WHY
MIXED FEEDING
MATTERS

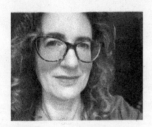

About the author

Karen Hall has been an NCT Breastfeeding Counsellor since 2009. She lives in Berkshire with her civil partner and their teenager. She is passionate about supporting parents to feed their babies, and loves communicating about feeding as well as other parenting topics.

For five years, she co-presented the popular podcast *Sprogcast*, and has gone on to make *The Breastfeeding Show* and *The Second Shift*. This is her first venture into writing a book, and she hopes it will add to her work as another useful, accessible resource for parents and birth workers alike.

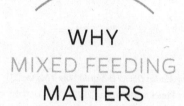

WHY
MIXED FEEDING
MATTERS

Karen Hall

pinter
&
martin

Why Mixed Feeding Matters (Pinter & Martin Why It Matters 25)

First published by Pinter & Martin Ltd 2023

©2023 Karen Hall

Karen Hall has asserted her moral right to be identified as the author of this work in accordance with the Copyright, Designs and Patents Act of 1988.

ISBN 978-1-78066-660-0

Also available as an ebook

Pinter & Martin Why It Matters ISSN 2056-8657

Series editor: Susan Last
Index: Helen Bilton
Cover Design: Blok Graphic, London
British Library Cataloguing-in-Publication Data

A catalogue record for this book is available from the British Library.

Set in Minion

Printed and bound in the UK by Clays

This book has been printed on paper that is sourced and harvested from sustainable forests and is FSC accredited.

Pinter & Martin Ltd
Unit 803 Omega Works
4 Roach Road
London E3 2PH

pinterandmartin.com

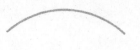

Contents

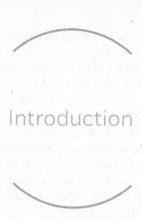

Introduction

Much of the conversation about feeding babies is centred around breastfeeding or bottle-feeding, as though each is completely exclusive of the other. Although it goes against guidelines, new mothers and parents-to-be are often asked, very early in pregnancy, which side they have picked. Opposing influences will then seek to persuade them over to the other side. All of this ignores the statistical fact that the most common way to feed a baby in the UK in the 21st century is with a mixture of breastmilk and formula milk. Sometimes this is a deliberate and positive decision, and sometimes it is a route that parents would not have chosen, but they felt that they had no alternative. Whichever pathway they have been on, many parents say that they feel unprepared for the realities of mixed feeding, unsupported, and often disappointed with their experience.

According to the 2010 Infant Feeding Survey[1] the initiation rate of breastfeeding in the UK at that time was 81%. At six weeks, 21% of babies were still exclusively fed on breastmilk, and 55% of babies were still getting some breastmilk, indicating a high rate of partial breastfeeding, whether this was the original plan or not. The same research tells us that of those mothers who had completely stopped breastfeeding by this time, 8 out of 10 had planned to breastfeed for longer, and often had feelings of grief and trauma associated with the disappointment of having to make this decision.[2] In the interests of optimising breastfeeding, and the overall experience, for those mothers or chestfeeding parents who are still giving any breastmilk at all at this stage, support and information should be readily available to help them to continue, or to change that situation when they feel ready. This is why mixed feeding matters.

You might have picked this book up before your baby is born, hoping for some ideas that will help you to make decisions about how you will feed your baby. You might be interested in breastfeeding, but worried that it won't work out for you, or that your partner will feel left out if you are doing all the feeding, or anxious for some other reason. Having a baby, and feeding a baby, are transformational experiences[3] – you might not know yet how becoming a parent will change you – and it can be hard to give you information that, at this stage, will feel meaningful to you. This is why I will share lots of parents' perspectives on their own experiences, so you can hear about it from people who are right in the middle of the process themselves, like this:

'In our antenatal class, lots of us asked about mixed feeding, but it felt like the subject was glossed over.' Anon

Remember, you don't actually have to make a decision yet: things could go in unexpected directions.

You might have picked this book up searching for practical guidance, having already made the decision to give your baby formula milk alongside breastmilk, whether that was a deliberate decision, or a situation that has developed and leaves you feeling like you don't have a choice. Either way, I hope this book will be helpful. I aim to include the practical information that you might need in a range of different situations, and also help you to explore your feelings about your decision.

Or you might be a midwife, health visitor, or someone else whose role is to support new families with their feeding decisions. There's not very much out there for you, so I'll try to offer some practical ideas and resources that you can use, as well as plenty of great signposts. Parents decide to mix-feed in so many different circumstances that it is not possible to take a one-size-fits-all approach, but there are skills you can bring to your role that will help you to be supportive and kind, whatever the situation.

Infant feeding in 21st-century Britain

Breastfeeding is a very well-researched area, but most investigations focus on health outcomes, duration, and support, with a basic assumption that the goal is exclusive breastfeeding. There isn't very much research that looks at parents' expectations and experiences of using both breastmilk and formula milk, despite this being such a common way to feed a baby in 21st-century Britain.

In the antenatal period, when infant feeding is all a bit abstract, parents-to-be often make two contradictory assumptions: first, that breastfeeding is 'all or nothing',[4] and second that if they can use a combination of breastmilk and formula, this will be easier than just breastfeeding, but better for their baby than just using formula.[5] This idea that you must choose one or the other plays into and perpetuates the divisive narrative pitching breastmilk against formula milk, and the idea that parents on each side must be judging those on the other side.[6] Meanwhile, those parents-to-be have also been informed by friends, family, and the media, that breastfeeding is hard, often doesn't work for unpredictable and uncontrollable reasons, and isn't very important anyway, suggesting that the introduction of a bottle of formula, at some point, is inevitable.

This is all very confusing. No wonder parents have such mixed feelings, and so often feel practically and emotionally unprepared and unsupported, whatever decisions they make.[2] This book sets out to share some of the experiences of new parents, some useful information to assist with decision-making, and plenty of ideas about who can offer support without judgement.

What do we mean by 'mixed feeding'?

In this book, we are talking about any situation where a baby is being given some breastmilk, alongside formula milk. This may also include expressed breastmilk (EBM) or donated human milk, which can sometimes be obtained from a local or national milk bank, or through informal milk sharing.

For any amount of the mother's own milk to be given to the baby, there needs to be an understanding of how breastfeeding works, so I will dedicate one chapter to establishing a milk supply and getting started. There are many good books on this, as well as videos, helplines, support groups, and antenatal classes. I'll let you know all about those.

When it comes to what you need to know about formula milk, it can be hard to find accurate information that comes without commercial influences. So I will give you the information you need to choose a suitable milk, prepare it safely for your baby, and offer it to them in an appropriately responsive way.

Who am I?

I am an NCT Breastfeeding Counsellor, with many years' experience of working with parents in antenatal classes and offering postnatal support, in a huge variety of different feeding situations. Breastfeeding Counsellors know how often parents-to-be ask about mixed feeding, and share their frustration in sometimes not being able to give very clear answers. This is often because there is very little research specifically about the experience of mixed feeding, and we don't like to make things up! It's also because parents mix-feed for so many different reasons, and in so many different situations, that there isn't very much we can say, antenatally, that would be helpful once they find themselves having to make the decisions in real time. What we do offer is kind, non-judgemental support, and a huge number of the families we help in the post-birth period are using formula milk alongside breastfeeding. If we are speaking to them, it is usually because they want to change the situation they're in at the time, and our job is to support them with the changes they are hoping to make.

I am also a mother of one, now a teenager, who presented all sorts of feeding challenges in the first months of their life. This is what motivated me to train as a Breastfeeding Counsellor, a life-changing and very rewarding decision. I have worked as a Parent Supporter for Netmums, and I've been making podcasts for many years too, which means I've had the chance to speak to many people with knowledge and perspectives that have informed this book. I also tutor for NCT, training the Breastfeeding Counsellors who will work and volunteer for the charity in the future.

A note about language

Mixed feeding is sometimes known as partial breastfeeding or combination feeding. I will use the term mixed feeding, as that is the one most commonly used by parents.

I have tried to use a variety of terms, including women, mothers, parents, families, breastfeeding and chestfeeding, to acknowledge transgender and gender non-conforming people who also have to make decisions about, and access support with, feeding their babies.

So why do parents decide to use a combination of breastmilk and formula?

> 'Everyone we know who has done the same have for different reasons and in different ways.' Charlotte

Parents do this for so many reasons, sometimes planned before the birth, often as a back-up, and too often it happens before they feel ready. This book is intended to offer information that might help with both the decision-making and the practicalities involved in this very common way to feed a baby. It is written with love to all the parents who find such decision-making difficult, and who have mixed feelings about how they are feeding their baby.

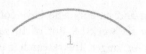

Why do parents use both breastmilk and formula?

In this chapter, I'm going to explore the social and cultural context of parental decisions to use both breastmilk and formula. If you're not here for the politics, do feel free to skip on to the more practical chapters later in the book. We are going to be looking at the role of the formula industry in shaping parents' expectations of feeding, and how the reality of life with a new baby can be quite different from what parents anticipate and looked forward to. This is to provide some context about how we make feeding decisions, and certainly not to suggest that anyone is doing it wrong.

What do we know about parents' intentions?

In my introduction, I mentioned the statistic that 81% of new mothers plan to breastfeed, and that at six weeks 21% of babies are exclusively breastfed, while 55% are getting some breastmilk. There is no research telling us the proportion of parents that planned to use both breastmilk and formula milk right from the start, but we do know that within the large group of women and parents who have completely stopped breastfeeding by six weeks, 9 out of 10 say that they had planned to do it for longer. The research is unclear about the plans or percentages of the women who are using both at this stage.

What we do know is that there is a fairly small group of parents who make a deliberate decision to start mixed feeding in those first six weeks, and a larger group of parents who find themselves using formula alongside breastfeeding, where this was not their original plan.

In the first group, those who make a deliberate decision do so for a range of different reasons, whether that is an instinctive sense that this is just the right thing for them, a decision made out of anxiety that breastfeeding won't work, or existing knowledge that exclusive breastfeeding is not a possibility. Some parents plan to breastfeed but also introduce a bottle (whether of formula or breastmilk) early on, in the expectation that this will make it easier to share feeding later.

'I wanted to share parenting and I didn't want to feel tied that I couldn't leave the baby. Therefore it was important that our baby took a bottle for an evening feed.' Marie

In the second group, we have another set of reasons, with breastfeeding not going well being right at the top of that list. There are also situations where a baby is not well enough to breastfeed, or the mother and baby might be separated. There can be pressures arising from lack of sleep, work, and family relationships, which lead to the introduction of formula milk.

'We introduced formula from the first day, because of lack of support with breastfeeding at hospital. I had an emergency c-section, and my arms were numb after the

epidural, so I couldn't breastfeed immediately after the surgery. My son got some hand-expressed colostrum but I was then left on my own, and it was only hours later at night that a midwife showed me how to breastfeed. By that point my baby was very hungry and I was exhausted after two days without sleep; I felt I had no choice but to give him formula to settle him. The next day I had severe side effects from the c-section and was put on morphine. My nipples were bleeding but again I had no help to breastfeed (despite asking for support), so my partner had to take over the feeds. I tried to express manually as much as I could, but the baby needed more, so we felt we had to use formula. We found it very difficult after that to go back to breastmilk only, as my milk production seemed always lower than our son's needs. I only received breastfeeding support (from the NCT) after I left the hospital on day four. My son is now 11 weeks and gets about half of his feed with formula.' Agi

'I had some sleepless nights and needed help. The first month of breastfeeding is so very challenging and I under-estimated how difficult it would be on me emotionally and physically.' Stephanie

In both groups, the decision to use some formula milk can give rise to a range of emotions: relief, guilt, and sadness among them. The decision can lift one burden and add another. There are often new and unpredictable challenges that arise from taking this new direction, and I will try to give you some information and ideas that will help.

'It was both a relief and a burden. I felt both like I was failing her and that I was doing the best that I could for

15

her. I felt unsupported but also that I hadn't done enough to find the support I needed. I felt that many friends and family were relieved that I started using formula and I resented them.' Frankie

The social and cultural context

Breastfeeding rates vary enormously around the world, with very high numbers of women exclusively breastfeeding at six months in parts of Scandinavia, and in many developing countries.[1] The USA and UK trail far behind, sharing the dubious accolade of having the world's lowest rates of exclusive breastfeeding at six months. This situation is self-perpetuating: the less breastfeeding there is, the less it is understood and valued in that society.

150 years ago, it would not have been controversial to state that breastfeeding was the optimal way to feed a baby, and since then an enormous body of research has continued to show that, on many measures, this is true.[2] The one thing that has changed, perhaps, is our understanding of what is 'optimal.' Over the last 150 years our way of life has been transformed: women expect to work outside the home, their partners expect to have an active role in parenting, and we do now have a safe and suitable alternative food for babies. And yet we are riddled, as a society, with contradictory assumptions. There is a reasonably good understanding of the positive health outcomes of breastfeeding, but alongside this a generalised expectation that it is difficult. Antenatally, parents tell me they will try it, and often add that they won't 'beat themselves up' if it doesn't work out.

'I said I'd give breastfeeding a go, see how it went.' Hester

Between the 1950s and 1970s, in the UK, breastfeeding initiation rates sank to 20–30% of new mothers.[3] The percentage began to creep up in the 1980s, and is currently around 80%. This increase happened because of various initiatives like the WHO International Code of Marketing of Breast-milk Substitutes,[4] which aims to protect parents, whether they are breastfeeding or bottle-feeding (or both), from inaccurate information about formula milk. This means that health professionals are less influenced by the manufacturers of formula milk, and that those manufacturers have to work harder to advertise to parents subtly enough not to contravene the Code.

And work hard they do. In fact, the formula industry spends £36 per baby on advertising in the UK,[5] and advertising is aimed directly at those parents who have made at least a tentative decision to breastfeed (because there is no need to advertise to those who have already decided to use their products).

> *'The majority of women come to using formula milk from breastfeeding. Therefore formula companies want to be linked with breastfeeding.'* Elizabeth Mayo, UNICEF BFI

This hard work includes offering breastfeeding support, providing sponsorship for health professionals' training and social media/celebrity/influencers' endorsements, creating products that circumvent the legislation about advertising, and producing adverts that idealise breastfeeding. Actually, this last one sounds great, doesn't it? If the formula industry explicitly tells us that breast is best, surely they must be the good guys? And yet suggesting that breastfeeding is ideal implies that it is an aspirational goal; normal parents, 'good enough' parents, use formula. Perpetuating the culture war between parents who breastfeed and parents who use formula means that the concept of breastfeeding as a lifestyle choice that is simply not for everyone persists. Parents absorb the message that bottles and formula are the cultural norm through social media, both explicitly (@nhsengland on Twitter used a row of bottle icons to congratulate the Duke and Duchess of Suffolk on the birth of their first child) and in more insidious ways, via the algorithms and cookies that follow us around the internet.

All this is to say, that many parents hope or plan to breastfeed, while also expecting to use formula from an early stage. Those breastfeeding hopes are often dashed early on, and we will shortly look at why that happens. Meanwhile the divisive narrative of breast v bottle gives rise to feelings of failure and disappointment, and often parents do not feel supported or prepared as they embark on mixed feeding, whether they have made a positive decision to do so, or feel that they have had it foisted upon them.

> *'My husband and family were very supportive. I found that all healthcare institutions make out that breast is best and push the topic to the point where you feel guilty for not exclusively breastfeeding.'* Grace

Health outcomes from breastfeeding

Researchers at Staffordshire University[6] found that some assumptions behind parents' decisions to mixed feed are based on misinformation, specifically that formula milk is nutritionally equivalent or even superior to breastmilk, and that breastfeeding is only beneficial in the short term.

A systematic review of the research, undertaken in 2016,[1] shows both of these assumptions to be incorrect. The authors summarised a huge body of research to show that breastfeeding has a protective effect against childhood infections including respiratory infections and diarrhoea, and non-communicable diseases such as type-2 diabetes, dental malocclusion, sudden infant death syndrome (SIDS), obesity, allergies and asthma. In addition, women who breastfed had a lower risk of breast and ovarian cancer, and type-2 diabetes, particularly when they breastfed for longer.

I would argue that most of the parents I have supported do not make decisions about whether or not to start or continue to breastfeed, on the basis of the health outcomes for themselves or their children, given the huge complexity and many factors involved in feeding decisions. Nonetheless, this information is important if you are going to make a fully informed decision. And remember that if you are mixed feeding, your baby is still having breastmilk: this is not an all-or-nothing situation.

Introducing formula milk before you had planned to

'At the start, we felt we had no other choice, and we thought it would be temporary for a few days, so we didn't think much about it. But later on when I realised that my milk production was never going to catch up (after weeks of pumping and breastfeeding 10 times a day), I was very disappointed and felt guilty that we let this happen.' Agi

Early supplements of formula can be suggested for all sorts of reasons, and parents do often feel as though they have little choice. Obviously babies need to be fed, and formula exists precisely for those situations where there is no other alternative. Please remember that, even when it feels like you are running out of options, seeking support may help you to make a decision you feel happy with. Your midwife should be able to refer you to an infant feeding midwife (with specialist skills and knowledge), or you could call a breastfeeding helpline or speak to a breastfeeding counsellor at a group.

Anxiety about breastfeeding

For a huge number of reasons, some of which I've touched on in the section above, many people worry about breastfeeding. This could be because of a family history or stories from friends about breastfeeding difficulties; previous trauma or abuse; body dysphoria; or the cumulative effect of the cultural attitude that breastfeeding just doesn't work for most people. In Scandinavia, 99% of babies are still breastfed at six months of age, which means it is not women's bodies that are at fault: rather, in 21st-century Britain, breastfeeding is not understood or valued, and this creates a self-perpetuating situation where the decision to breastfeed is difficult to sustain.

'I intended to breastfeed if I could…' Samira

'Breastfeeding if possible but open to formula if needed.' Louise

'I planned on exclusively breastfeeding if I could.' Stephanie

'I had formula ready in case I didn't produce any milk.' Claire

An individual's confidence in breastfeeding can be fragile, and at the first sign of things not going well, formula milk is often offered. We will look in Chapter 6 at how this can be done without undermining breastfeeding, but it is often the case that this is not well managed.

Planning to use both breastmilk and formula milk from the start or in the early days

Whether for pragmatic reasons or from anxiety, some parents know that they intend to introduce formula very early in their baby's life, and plan to combine breastmilk and formula for at least several weeks. In some cases, this can go on for months, and in Chapter 6 we are going to discuss some ways to sustain this situation in the longer term.

> *'I did this with my son because it took us ages to get going with breastfeeding and my milk didn't seem to come in as fast as it had done with my daughter, in the end I fed him until he was almost one.'* Hester

There are some cultural assumptions at play here, particularly the idea that babies sleep better on formula, and that a breastfeeding lifestyle can be stressful, chaotic, and an uneven burden on the breastfeeding (or chestfeeding) parent.

Expectations of newborn sleep

It's a very common experience to be asked by friends, family, and even complete strangers, whether your newborn is a 'good' baby. You will be unsurprised to learn that they are not asking whether they seem inclined towards a career in bank robbery or politics, but that in fact they are trying to find out if the baby sleeps much. The Victorian notion that a good baby is one who sleeps for long stretches has been repeatedly debunked, and in fact the opposite has been proven: it is good for babies to wake repeatedly throughout the day and night.[7]

A 2012 review of the research[8] showed that newborn sleep has a huge range, with some babies sleeping for a total of 8–12 hours out of 24, and others sleeping 22–24 hours out of 24, generally with no ill effects. Babies have a very small stomach capacity (about the size of a cherry), and digest their milk quickly, which means they need frequent refills. Milk at this stage is growing the brain as much as the body, and those frequent wakings mean babies also benefit from repeated interaction and touch from their caregivers, which again stimulates brain growth. A normal newborn sleep cycle will tend to be shorter and lighter than that of an adult, and any time the baby wakes, if she or he does not at that point feel safe and comfortable, they will 'signal' to their caregiver for help. In other words, when they wake up, they need the attention of an adult to help them get back to sleep. For more on normal newborn sleep, I can recommend the Baby Sleep Info Source website, from the University of Durham (www.basisonline.org.uk).

In the developed western world, we associate sleep and feeding very closely,[9] meaning that if sleep is perceived by parents to be an issue, then it doesn't take long for the focus to become the feeding. Parents-to-be will be told by friends, family and the media that the solution to this perceived problem is to give a bottle of formula at night. This is thought to be helpful in one (or both) of two ways: firstly, it is thought that babies sleep more soundly if given formula; and secondly, if someone else can give a bottle, then the mother can take a longer break between feeds and therefore get more rest. We will look at the latter idea in more detail in Chapter 6, as there are some things to consider in order to get the desired benefits. The idea that babies will sleep more soundly after a bottle of formula also needs to be explored.

This may well have been true a few decades ago, but the composition of modern formula has improved such that it is more easily digested than early formulas. More importantly, perhaps, we parent differently now. Historically, it was generally considered that formula-fed babies woke less frequently at night, but this was at a time when babies were likely to sleep separately from their parents, on their fronts, and it was more common to give large bottle feeds less frequently.[10] All of these factors (sleeping in a separate room, sleeping on their front, not breastfeeding) are likely to cause babies to sleep more soundly and are also associated with a higher risk of cot death, properly known as Sudden Infant Death Syndrome (SIDS), and the first two are now actively discouraged by Safer Sleep guidelines (see www.lullabytrust.org). Rates of SIDS have dramatically decreased as a result, but the belief that babies who have formula milk will sleep longer persists. There are now quite a few studies showing either no overall difference,[11] or that mothers who breastfeed at night get the same amount[12] or even more sleep[13] than those who do not.

To unpick the belief that formula-fed babies sleep longer a little further we can think about 'regression to the mean'. This is the statistical concept that if you take two samples (e.g. baby's sleep last night, baby's sleep tonight), an extreme point will usually be followed by a less extreme point. In other words, parents may assume that the actions they took tonight (e.g. giving a bottle of formula) are the cause of the better sleep. Since they are more likely to give that bottle when the situation reaches an intolerable extreme, regression to the mean tells us that the baby may well have had a better night the next night regardless of the bottle.

'Initially I wanted to do the one bottle of formula to give myself a break and was also told that formula before bed helps baby sleep better.' Grace

None of this is to say that you should not give a bottle, but it won't necessarily guarantee you a good night's sleep. Babies wake for reasons other than hunger, and having a range of coping strategies at your disposal is always going to be helpful. And give yourself a break:

'The measure of how "good" a parent you are is not how "well" your child sleeps'. Lyndsey Hookway, *Let's Talk About Your New Family's Sleep.*[14]

Transition to parenthood

It is impossible to really know what parenthood will be like before you experience it. Some people may have spent time close to a family, or had numerous younger siblings, but it is still very difficult to understand the push and pull of parenthood: it is possible to want to spend every moment gazing at your child, and at the same time to be crying out for a break and some time to yourself.[15] In pregnancy, we imagine the kind of parents we will be, and take on board all manner of advice about retaining your identity and making sure the baby isn't the boss of you. I can vividly remember some acquaintances, an older couple, repeatedly advising me to make sure that we 'got out as a couple' at the earliest opportunity. My childless sister-in-law wanted to take me out and make me feel like 'one of the girls' again. What I actually felt like was someone who no longer spoke the same language or lived in the same time zone as other people. Gone were my predictable, structured work life, regular meals, weekend lie-ins, and even any control over my day-to-day existence.

'I was thinking about introducing formula at the six-week mark, so my husband could help with feeds once breastfeeding was established, and I could have some freedom to get out without the time pressure.' Stephanie

It may feel as though having the option of giving formula milk will give you back some of this control, whether that's providing you with a break, or imposing a little bit of routine on newborn chaos. This works for some families; but for others it adds in extra stress. In Chapter 6 we will explore ways of doing it.

Wanting the other parent to be involved

> '*We are members of the exclusive club of 5 per cent of mammal species – and the only ape – whose males invest in their offspring.*' Anna Machin, *The Life of Dad*

I was born in 1970. My dad was in the pub with his mates at the time, but visited me later that day (he says he was euphoric; I expect he'd had a Guinness or two). Mum stayed in hospital for a week. Eighteen years later my dad was present at my half-sister's birth. Over a couple of decades, western society's expectations of new fathers had completely changed. Half a century ago, the role of the father was pretty clear: man hunter-gatherer, man provide. Families now are far less constrained by gender roles, heteronormativity, and convention. Despite this, the narrative persists that the non-breastfeeding partner will feel 'left out' of the relationship between breastfeeding parent and child, and the breastfeeding parent will be excessively burdened by the sole responsibility of keeping the baby alive.

> '*We had planned to stick to breastmilk, but wanted to introduce bottle-feeding from the start so that the father could be involved in the feeds.*' Agi

> '*It did make it easier because others could formula feed and baby wasn't reliant on just me.*' Samira

This idea of the 'involved father' or 'New Dad' emerged in the 1980s. Rather similarly to the mum who can 'have it all', New Dad gets to win bread *and* change nappies! Breastfeeding is idealised as, among other things, a beautiful bonding experience, with the implication that parents who don't breastfeed will bond less, or take longer to form an attachment with their child. In fact, the process of forming an attachment, like the growth of any relationship, will be affected by a whole range of factors, but particularly the amount of time spent interacting with one another. Baby care offers lots of opportunities for interaction: newborns love to watch faces and listen to voices, and will enjoy the familiarity of seeing and hearing their close carers. Babies sleep much better in contact with human beings, and that contact can be provided by other adults than the breastfeeding mother. Bath time can be lots of fun, and it's never too early to read to your child – really, any sort of interaction with the baby helps to develop that relationship.

> 'A father is the first person to teach his baby that love doesn't have to come with food.' Anne Altshuler, RN, MS, IBCLC, LLL Leader[16]

Meanwhile, a mother recovering from birth and trying to establish breastfeeding is likely to need some support. She may be tired, sore, tearful, and a bit overwhelmed by all that she feels she has to do. A partner who can be present for this, practically and emotionally, is doing a lot to ease her way through this challenging time. In *The Life of Dad* (2018), Anna Machin[17] writes that a key factor in how well a father bonds with his child is the strength of his relationship with his partner. This looks like a win-win: by caring for the new mother so that she can care for the baby, the new dad is strengthening his relationship with both of them.

We'll come back to this in Chapter 5 to suggest some ways that giving a bottle might work, if this feels particularly important to you for this reason. But do consider the many other ways partners can interact with the baby, and support the new mother, in addition to giving that bottle of milk.

Cultural practices

Breastfeeding doesn't look the same everywhere. In certain cultures, colostrum is not given to the baby because it is considered dirty or stale, as it has been in the breast since before the baby was born. The baby would instead be given different things in different cultures, but often something sweet like honey, sweetened tea, or formula. This does not necessarily mean that the mother does not intend to breastfeed, but it is worth being mindful that a delayed start to breastfeeding can make it harder to get started.

There are also many situations where mixed feeding enables a woman to be part of society, where she cannot or does not want to breastfeed in public or in front of men. Expressed milk or formula are both options, and we will look later in the book at how to balance these with continued breastfeeding.

Medical conditions that can make it difficult to establish a full milk supply

Confusingly, you may have heard either that all women can breastfeed, or that many women just can't, or even have been told both at some point! In truth, studies show that an inability to produce breastmilk for purely physiological reasons occurs in 2–5% of the population.[18]

The most common medical conditions that affect a woman's ability to produce a full supply of milk are diabetes, PCOS, untreated thyroid conditions, retained placenta, and major blood loss during the birth. The latter two will usually resolve over time, and in all the above cases, skilled breastfeeding support can make a difference.

Insufficient Glandular Tissue (IGT), also known as hypoplasia or hypoplastic breast syndrome, is a rare condition in which milk-producing glands do not develop in the breast during puberty. Women or parents with this condition usually find that although colostrum is produced, mature milk does not develop in a sufficient quantity for full breastfeeding. With good support and an effective latch, some breastfeeding should be possible, and sometimes the galactagogues mentioned in Chapter 6 can help, but this is one of those situations where mixed feeding might be hard to avoid.

'I wish someone would acknowledge that I didn't have enough milk rather than telling me continuously that every mum has enough milk and baby would be fine. Baby was very irritable and cried constantly for her first three months of life and I believe that was because she was hungry and wasn't getting enough from me. Healthcare professionals weren't prepared to admit that.' Anna

Some breast surgery can restrict the ability to produce a full supply of milk, but because milk ducts can regrow, it will depend on the nature of the surgery. This is often a 'wait and see' situation, where you will not know how much breastfeeding is possible until you start doing it. The website bfar.org is extremely useful and has a supportive community attached.

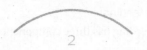

2

What do parents need to know about breastfeeding?

Without a supply of breastmilk, mixed feeding is never going to be a realistic possibility. In the absence of any breastfeeding issues, the guidance is generally to get this established first, if this is possible, as it will tend to make things more straightforward. The production of breastmilk relies on milk being removed from the breast, so to meet your baby's needs this does need to be happening, whether by direct breastfeeding, expressing, or a combination of both. Once some formula is introduced, the supply of breastmilk will usually decrease, which is necessary, as an oversupply of milk can be uncomfortable and sometimes leads to mastitis.

In this section, we're going to look at what's happening in the new mother's body, alongside what the baby is likely to be doing, and how these two factors work together to help get breastfeeding started. In chapters 5 and 6 we will then look at how you might tip the balance towards either more or less breastfeeding, managing the supply of breastmilk according to your needs.

Effective breastfeeding

Effective breastfeeding has three components:

- Early feeding
- Frequent feeding
- Deep attachment (latch)

We'll explore all of these things as we go along, starting at the very beginning.

Colostrum

The first substance the mother produces is called colostrum. This is usually yellowish in colour, thicker than milk, and contains among other things a range of important antibodies, as well as growth factors such as hormones and protein. It is usually produced from around 17–22 weeks of pregnancy, and some women notice this more than others. In some parts of the UK, midwives are keen to encourage pregnant women to try to collect some colostrum before the baby is born. The reason for doing this is as a back-up plan, in case for any reason the baby doesn't feed in the first few hours after birth, which is when small amounts of formula are sometimes offered. Research shows that those early formula feeds can make it more difficult to get breastfeeding started,[1,2] hence the move towards offering small amounts of expressed colostrum instead. This could be expressed before the birth (midwives usually suggest from 36 weeks of pregnancy), or it could be expressed at the time it is needed. Colostrum is usually expressed by hand rather than with a pump. There's a handy video that one of my colleagues made, which shows you how to go about this, at www.facebook.com/watch/?v=242126123722025.

You will need a few tiny 1ml colostrum syringes, which

your midwife should give you at your last appointment before 36 weeks. It's worth bearing in mind that not everyone finds it easy to express colostrum, and yet pretty much everyone is producing it by the last weeks of pregnancy. If it's not coming out for you, please don't panic – that doesn't mean it isn't there. You may well have more success once your baby is born and you can spend time with them, hopefully cuddling them, gazing at them, and letting the oxytocin flow.

Some people worry that expressing colostrum in advance will mean that they don't have enough left when the baby is born. Happily this isn't how it works, as we will see when we look at milk supply in the next section.

Hormones and milk supply

One of the biggest things that new parents worry about is having enough milk to feed the baby. I'm going to explain the science here, and later on give you some ideas about how you can monitor feeding to reassure yourself that it is going well. If you'd rather have an analogy, think of the system as a river, not a reservoir: milk isn't stored in the breast until needed, but produced as and when it is required.

A mother's supply of breastmilk is driven by the action of one main hormone, called *prolactin* (which if you know Latin you'll recognise as meaning 'for milk'). Prolactin is released by the pituitary gland in response to milk being removed from the breast (i.e. by a baby feeding or a mother expressing milk). It triggers prolactin receptors in the breast, causing the milk glands to produce milk. This is a complicated way of saying that when milk is removed from the breast, the breast produces more milk.

This is not the same as saying that the more your baby feeds, the more milk you produce, which is only true if the baby is feeding effectively: frequently, and with a good latch.

More on this shortly.

Breastmilk also contains a protein called *feedback inhibitor of lactation* (FIL), which signals to the brain that milk is no longer needed. So if milk is allowed to build up (e.g. there is a long gap between feeds), then FIL also builds up, causing production to stop. If milk is frequently removed, FIL is only present in small quantities, and therefore production continues. This is a complicated way of saying that an emptier breast makes milk more quickly than a full breast.

Oxytocin also has an important role in breastfeeding. You may know this hormone from such conversations as 'how to help a woman's body to push a baby out', and 'that squishy feeling of being in love'. Oxytocin is a multi-tasking hormone that supports bonding, helps to regulate physiological systems such as circulation and temperature control, produces the contractions needed to birth the baby, and in breastfeeding oxytocin is what releases the milk. If you've done an antenatal course you may have had some discussion of how to elevate oxytocin levels to assist with birth; these same ideas are going to be useful in breastfeeding, assisted by the closeness and contact you will inevitably have with your baby, and some kind, loving support from those around you. If oxytocin causes the breast to release milk, then stress may work against this. It's also worth considering the role of oxytocin when expressing milk: a breast pump may not elicit that same squishy feeling of being in love that you get when cuddling your baby, and therefore the milk may not be so readily released – so it's particularly important to get your oxytocin-enhancing strategies in place when expressing, especially if you seem to be doing it under pressure.

For much more on oxytocin, you could look at the work of researcher Kerstin Uvnäs Moberg,[3] who has written several books and articles about it.

Summary

Frequent effective feeding → increased prolactin → milk is produced

Milk builds up → FIL builds up → milk production stops

Calm, relaxed environment → increased oxytocin → milk is released

What happens when the baby is born?

We know that the mother's body is already producing colostrum, and she may have noticed this or even collected some in advance of the birth. Prolactin increases during pregnancy, causing changes within the breast such as the growth of milk ducts, but the presence of the pregnancy hormone progesterone prevents the body from starting to make milk. When the baby is born and the placenta leaves the woman's body, thereby removing the source of the pregnancy hormones, milk production will begin. Prolactin levels remain high if the baby continues to feed. If not, they will gradually drop, and so will the production of milk.

Over the next three or four days, the quantity of milk produced will increase, and the composition will change. Many mothers find that somewhere between days three and five, there's a noticeable change in the amount of milk, and the breasts may become very heavy and tender (engorged). This may be accompanied by a period of low mood, tears, and a need for wine/chocolate/kind empathic support. This feeling will usually pass.

With regard to the engorgement that occurs when the milk changes, this can make it more difficult for the baby to latch on, as the breast is likely to be bigger and firmer than before. Sometimes it helps to express a little bit just before feeding, to soften the breast, so the baby can latch on more easily. It might be an idea to save that milk in the fridge, and put the baby to the breast so they can get on with stimulating the milk supply and refining their innate breastfeeding skills. You could also try something called 'reverse pressure softening,' which is gentle pressure around the areola to relieve swelling and soften the breast to make it easier for the baby to latch on. There are good instructions for this here: kellymom.com/bf/ concerns/mother/rev_pressure_soft_cotterman/

How much and how often?

One of the downsides of breasts is the absence of a small meter on the side to indicate how much milk is available and how much has been removed. We are going to look at how you can tell it's working in more detail, but one of the good signs is simply that the baby's feeding pattern fits into the range of normal.

When we're talking about human behaviour, of course there is always a range. Perhaps it would help to think about how often you eat and drink during a 24-hour period, and if you have someone nearby you can ask them the same question. Do you both come up with the same number? Probably not. Now consider whether every time you ate or drank, it was purely to satisfy hunger or thirst? Perhaps there were some other things going on: you might have a cool refreshing drink because it's a hot day, or how about a nice cup of tea? Maybe you shared a piece of cake with a visitor. Or if you're really lucky, you were out for a lovely romantic meal, with candlelight and soft music, all your favourite food, and the company of someone you love. Or you grabbed a biscuit from the tin just because it was there. Humans need connection, and much of our eating and drinking is tangled up in that need. When a baby feeds, they are also meeting all of those social and emotional needs, without ever being able to articulate exactly what it is that they want from you. Obviously this is true whether a baby is fed at the breast or with a bottle, or a bit of both, so bottle feeds can incorporate all of this loving contact as well.

Your baby is likely to need to feed somewhere between 10 and 14 times in 24 hours, with feeds lasting between 5 and roughly 45 minutes, although they might sometimes go on for longer (remember the romantic meal). You may have a baby with very consistent feeding behaviour, or one who likes to keep you guessing. If they are feeding effectively, then all you have to do is follow their lead.

Interestingly, babies are really good at regulating their milk intake, and this again is to do with oxytocin: at the start of a breastfeed, there is a build-up of milk in the breast. As the milk releases, it tends to flow quite quickly, and the particles of fat will adhere to the milk ducts, beginning to drop into the milk as the amount in the breast decreases. Therefore the fat content of the milk is gradually increasing through the feed, until it triggers an oxytocin response in the baby, and the baby stops feeding. When they stop, they may let go of the breast, or they might have fallen asleep with it in their mouth; if you gently release the latch and move them away, you'll soon know if they were hoping to stay there. This would be a good time to offer the second breast, which will be a little fuller, and so the milk available will be lower in fat, and the baby might take some more of it. At the next feed, start with the second breast from the previous feed. This allows the baby to continue regulating the volume and fat content of the milk, and reduces the likelihood of an excessive build-up of milk which can lead to blocked ducts or mastitis, and allow FIL to signal to the body that the milk is not needed (see above). This is not the case if the baby is getting his or her milk via a bottle, hence the importance of paced bottle feeding (see Chapter 5).

If you've had a go at collecting some colostrum, you might have noticed what tiny quantities we're talking about at the very start. Each feed at this stage is probably less than 5ml, increasing gradually over the days and weeks that follow, so that by the end of the month an exclusively breastfeeding mother might be producing a litre of milk over the course of the day. But to start with, you're looking at tiny amounts, the size of a grape or a full teaspoon. This is an appropriate amount for the newborn's tiny stomach capacity, which will also be increasing over the days and weeks that follow. When your baby is taking tiny amounts of a highly digestible fluid, they're going to need to do this over and over again in those first few days, and each time they feed, more prolactin is released, and the milk supply builds up a little further. Those 10–14 feeds in 24 hours start to make some sense now! Each time you feed your baby, you also meet that huge need for closeness and contact, and ease your baby's transition from the cosy safe world of the womb, to this outside world which, to start with, is so unfamiliar.

Feeding a newborn can be intense, time-consuming, and tiring. Those 10–14 feeds aren't likely to be evenly spaced and predictable; nor are they likely to fit neatly into daylight hours, or any time that feels particularly convenient for you. Some of them will melt together into what's known as a 'cluster feed', where you can't tell the end of one from the start of the next, and the baby is just not happy unless he or she is at the breast. Some babies will do this randomly, and some consistently.

Some babies will cluster feed in the early evening and then sleep like troopers;[4] others will find their feeding groove in the early hours of the morning. Whatever your baby tends to do, even completely normal newborn feeding can be hard work, so it may be helpful to consider what will help you get through this time. Here are some suggestions from parents who have recently been through it:

'Have some snacks by the bed – breastfeeding is hungry work!' Emma

'Set your bed up for safe sharing – once I'd stopped fighting the idea breastfeeding become much easier!' Jennifer

'I remember feeling incredibly guilty that my baby was waking often in the night as my husband had to work the following day. It transpired that my husband didn't mind a bit. Because he was at work all day he was grateful to spend time settling the little one in the night. So don't forget to communicate with your partner!' Nancy

'Have a water bottle instead of a glass of water, so you can't spill it!' Stacey

'My hubby does the night time change. So our routine is baby wakes up, hubby gets him up and changes him if he needs it whilst I get myself set up to breastfeed, he gives me baby then goes back to sleep. I feed and put baby back to bed.' Sarah

'Set up a breastfeeding "station" wherever you're feeding. Mine is a side table in the lounge next to my spot on the sofa because I pump after I've fed my daughter. Table

contains water, nipple cream, my book if I can stay awake enough to read and the remote control for when I really need to be kept awake! Oh, and a snack!' Rachel

'I had a little mantra – this will pass, they will sleep, this constant feeding will end, you've got this! Tried not to look at the clock and just appreciate every minute I could sleep.' Sarah

'If you've got an older child then have toys or games that you can play one-handed, or from the sofa! Eye spy, treasure hunts and tea parties are good ones.' Mel

'Go to bed as early as possible. My baby was a really bad sleeper both day and night, so for the first few months I would go to bed early (like 8pm) to gain as much sleep as possible.' Katie

'Bottle of water, and a travel mug so that your tea is still warm an hour later. Remember that the first three months is known as the fourth trimester, so if all you do is feed and change your baby, and the only place they will sleep is on you, they're just looking for what they know – you're their entire world.' Jen

'Have entertainment at the ready. A Kindle that lights up, audio books, or something to read/look at on your phone. Red light filters are a great help too (I use an app called Twilight). Just reduces the blue light from screens and should disrupt your body less so you can get back to sleep easier. Also, I learned this too late but I'd definitely recommend the Bluetooth headphones that come inside a stretchy headband. No wires to get tangled up in, not

disturbing anyone else and they're comfy for lying down in!' Hannah

'If you have a partner to help, getting them to do the lights, help you get comfortable etc really makes a difference in terms of emotional support. Lights – get a night light which is bright enough to help you sort out latch but not too much to wake everyone up loads.' Lotta

'A support network! My NCT group were amazing and I couldn't have done it without them. At your 4am feed when you're going crazy from exhaustion, sore as anything, knowing others are awake and you're all going through it together on your WhatsApp chat!' Kaval

'From a single mum perspective then def Netflix and a caddy by the bed with snacks, water bottle and baby bits. Get it all ready so you have everything for the night. Would just binge watch a show whilst feeding in the night, everytime he woke the glow of the TV was enough for me to see to feed and then I just continued watching my show and it kept me from falling asleep!' Anna

Some of these might work for you, and some won't fit your family situation.

Responding to your baby's cues

If you ask around – your granny, some old ladies at the bus stop, Twitter – 'How will I know when to feed my baby?' – you may well be advised to wait until they cry. Babies, however, are far more subtle and sophisticated in their communication than this might imply. If you've ever held a baby, you may have noticed them doing funny little movements with their head and particularly their mouth. These lip-smacking movements and the wide gaping mouth might look to you like things a baby would do if they wanted to latch on to the breast, and you would be right. The side-to-side head movements (known as 'rooting') enable a baby whose head is near the breast to find it using their own sense of smell, limited vision, and touch. So another answer to your question is, feed them when they do these things that will help them with the activity. A baby who is well supported, stable and comfortable against their mother's body, will often wriggle and push with their feet until they are in a position to root to the breast, open wide, and latch.

You don't have to wait for these signals though. With a newborn baby, you might offer a feed as soon as they seem to be stirring. At this stage, they will usually be calm, which means it is easier for them to coordinate their movements and find the breast. Holding your baby so that there is full contact between their body and yours will often release or trigger these movements: so much the better.

Feeding in response to these signals helps the mother's body to adjust the milk supply according to the baby's needs, as well as helping the baby to learn that their parents are reliable, kind people who are willing to meet their needs. No matter how much of a genius your child is, a newborn baby does not have the brain capacity to plan, which they would need to be able to manipulate you. Therefore, feeding the baby when they signal their need cannot possibly spoil them.

Do remember that babies usually feed between 10 and 14 times in 24 hours, and if your baby is not signalling that frequently, it might be helpful to feed them proactively, and to seek support from a breastfeeding counsellor or your midwife.

An effective latch

An effective latch means that the baby's mouth finds the breast and connects in a way that is comfortable for both the mother and the baby, and that transfers the milk from the breast to the baby. This is important for three main reasons:

1. As the baby removes milk, more milk is produced, so the breastmilk supply continues to meet the baby's needs.
2. The baby therefore gets the milk they need to support their growth.
3. It doesn't hurt, and therefore is sustainable for both the mother and the baby.

You will very often hear that people find breastfeeding painful, and I am not here to tell you that it should never hurt, or that if it does, you are doing it wrong. It's normal that things may feel a bit tender for the first few feeds, and usually more so at the start of a feed, with an intense sensation that usually settles down within a few seconds. However, when discomfort continues beyond the first few feeds, this is usually a sign that the latch is not effective. There is no point in pressing on through the pain, hoping to 'toughen up', or assuming that painful feeding is inevitable, because if the baby's latch is not effective, then they will be unlikely to take all the milk that they need, and this will result in less milk being produced. Treat any ongoing pain or discomfort as a red flag, signalling your need for some good quality breastfeeding support. Other signs of an ineffective latch could be that the nipple is misshapen (looking like the tip of a new lipstick, rather than rounded) or has changed colour from normal, when the baby lets go; or when the baby is unable to stay comfortably at the breast, and keeps slipping off.

There are some excellent videos on YouTube showing how the baby latches on, using a combination of animation and real footage. Search for Global Health Media's video 'Attaching your baby at the breast'.

For a comfortable latch, the baby's mouth needs to be very wide open, and positioned initially so that the nipple is roughly aligned with the baby's nose. If the baby is in a stable position, this usually encourages them to tilt their head back slightly, and gape their mouth very wide open.

To be in a stable position, it is often helpful if the mother can recline slightly, with the baby supported on her body (search 'laid back breastfeeding' or 'koala hold'). Remember that the heaviest part of the baby's body is their head, and when the baby is lying in the mother's arms, gravity will pull the head away from the breast. If the mother leans back and rests the baby on her own body, gravity does the opposite: it helps the baby to stay comfortably at the breast. For the baby, the environment of the mother's body usually feels safe and comfortable; full body contact stimulates feeding cues, which are behaviours like gaping, rooting/head-turning, and pushing with the feet and hands – all of these behaviours can usefully be coordinated to help the baby to latch on at the breast.

Breasts, as you may have noticed, are circular. This means that the baby can approach from any angle, and potentially latch on well. And this means that there is no 'correct' way to do this, so it is worth experimenting with different positions. Could lying down with your baby beside you on the bed work? Or curled up in a chair with the knees supporting the baby? The key is for the breastfeeding mother/chestfeeding parent to be sitting or lying in a stable, comfortable position, and then to bring the baby to the body.

It can be very helpful to seek support with this, from

someone with good credentials in supporting breastfeeding. All of the charities and their helplines are listed at the start Chapter 10 on p137. You may well have a local drop-in group at a Children's Centre, or run by your NCT branch, or a midwife-run clinic that you can attend. If face-to-face support is not available, many Breastfeeding Counsellors offer online support, and are also skilled at helping with positioning and attachment over the telephone.

How do I know it's working?

As we have said, there is no meter on the side of the breast to tell you how much milk the baby has taken. Even if there was, it would be very little help, because when a baby is feeding effectively they will self-regulate, and only take as much or as little as they need at each feed. It can be hard to trust a baby to do this, so it may be helpful to have some concrete signs that you can look out for.

1. Wet and dirty nappies

In the first hours after birth, the baby usually passes meconium: a black sticky poo that is made up of all the goo that is in their bowel at birth. This will change over the first two to three days, becoming more green and frothy, and decreasing in quantity. This green pesto-like stuff is the waste from colostrum, and it is a good sign. We mentioned above that the milk usually changes between three and five days, and as this happens, the poo will begin to change again, turning yellow and increasing in quantity. From this point onwards, you would expect to see a minimum of two dirty nappies in 24 hours, although many babies will do a lot more than this.

It can be hard to tell if the nappy is wet, especially with disposables, which are very effective at drawing moisture away from the surface. Some parents find it helpful to put a tissue in the nappy, so that there is evidence of wetness. In the first week, expect to see one wet nappy per day of life (one on day one, three on day three, etc). Thereafter, five to six wet nappies in 24 hours is about right.

2. Feeds are in the range of normal

As outlined above, if your baby feeds about 10–14 times in 24 hours, and the feeds last at least five minutes and generally not longer than 45 minutes to one hour, this is well within the range of normal. If there are many more, or many fewer feeds, or if they are shorter or regularly much longer than this, it would be a good idea to seek some support. This could be normal for your baby, but it helps to look at the bigger picture with someone objective and experienced.

3. Levels of alertness

Newborns can be sleepy, but will usually wake up frequently for feeds. While this can be relentless, it is necessary both for the baby to get the milk they need, and to stimulate milk production. A baby who is thriving will sleep, sometimes for 2–3 hours at a time (but often for less), but crucially, they will wake themselves up to feed, and they will usually have periods of alertness from time to time. Where a baby sleeps for very long periods (more than five hours at a time), it may be necessary to actively wake them to feed, but again, try to look at the big picture, including wet and dirty nappies, and frequency and length of feeds.

4. Weight gain

Weight gain is nice and measurable, which sometimes means we can have a tendency to focus on it and forget about items 1–3 above. It's common for babies to lose weight in the first few days of life, especially if the mother had intravenous fluids during labour. A weight loss of 5–7% of the birthweight is considered normal, and most babies will regain their birth weight by three weeks. After this, the NHS advises monthly weighing to check that they continue to grow at a healthy weight.[5]

When a baby continues to lose weight, or gains weight more slowly than expected, this is sometimes the point at which formula may be introduced. Chapters 5 and 6 will look at how you might manage this in order to stay on your preferred feeding journey.

Breastfeeding challenges

In the last few pages, I have mostly been talking about normal breastfeeding. The most common challenges arise when something appears to be outside this range of normal, and this can happen for a variety of reasons. It is always useful, at this point, to seek skilled breastfeeding support from someone who can listen to what's going on, and help you to explore how this fits with your expectations. It is very often the case that formula milk is introduced because of one or more of these challenging situations, with the two broad themes being concerns about the mother's supply of breastmilk (e.g. baby isn't gaining weight, feeds are very frequent, etc), or some version of the baby not latching on effectively, so that feeds are very painful for the mother, or hardly happening at all. Both of these themes will be addressed in Chapter 6 on managing breastfeeding alongside formula, and the range of support available to you is outlined in Chapter 10.

3

What do parents need to know about using formula milk?

Babies need breastmilk, formula, or a combination of the two, until they are one year old. In Chapter 1 we explored some of the statistics showing just how many babies in the UK are getting some formula, often in the early days, and almost always by six months. Several studies have found that parents feel unsupported and unprepared for using formula milk, and would like to have more information available to them, to help in their decision-making.[1,2,3] And yet there is some crucial information that parents need, so that their babies can have safe and appropriate food, on those occasions when they are not having breastmilk.

> *'Frantic searching on the internet. Was given a choice of formula on the paediatric ward but no information about it. Was just told to pick one'.* Simon

Parents get information about formula milk from friends and family, the NHS, online forums and social media, healthcare professionals, and from formula milk companies. Not all of these sources are robust or free of bias.

> *'A combination feeding group on Facebook gave me lots of help.'* Alex

Research from Swansea University in 2020[4] showed that the majority of parents have seen formula being advertised, and are familiar with claims that the product is 'advanced', or 'closest to breastmilk', or has special added ingredients. Breastmilk cannot be replicated because its composition changes at every feed, according to the needs of the baby. Formula milk exists so that babies who are not (always) getting breastmilk can have food that is safe for them to consume, and will support their growth and development. Parents need facts, not advertising slogans, to be able to choose the appropriate product from the overwhelming range that is available.

Safe and appropriate formula feeding

This has three components:

- Choosing the right milk
- Preparing it correctly
- Feeding responsively

Responsive feeding means picking up on and responding to your baby's feeding signals, as described in Chapter 2. We will come back to this in Chapter 5.

Choosing the right milk

There are four or five main manufacturers of formula milk, each of which has more than one brand, within which there are many, many different products. It is intentionally confusing. This is a lucrative industry, and regulations are weak. The regulations are there to protect parents from exploitation and misinformation, and the formula manufacturers work very hard at getting around them. This is not intended as a judgement of the product or those who use it. However, it is important that you have clear and accurate information about the different types of milk.

In 2019, Channel 4's *Dispatches*[5] programme revealed an alarming price differential between nutritionally equivalent products. At the time of writing, the First Steps Nutrition Trust[6] website compares prices per 100ml of ready-mixed liquid and made-up powdered formula, and some examples are shared here to show a comparison between the cheapest and the most expensive version of these nutritionally equivalent products:

Aptamil 1 First Milk starter pack (6 x 70ml)	274p
Aptamil 1 First Milk liquid (70ml carton)	60p
Aptamil 1 First Milk liquid (100ml)	43p
Aptamil 1 First Milk tablets	30p
Aptamil Advanced 1 First Milk powder	27p
Aptamil 1 First Milk powder	21p
Aldi Mamia First Infant Milk powder	12p

A higher price generally indicates added unnecessary ingredients and a greater marketing spend, but is certainly no indication of it being better for your baby.

Suitable from birth

The only type of milk suitable for your newborn baby is *first infant milk*. It should be clearly labelled 'suitable from birth', and usually has a big 1 on the side so that even the most sleep-deprived new parent can locate it on the supermarket shelf. This is the milk that is formulated according to a tightly regulated recipe (The Food for Specific Groups regulations, 2020), to meet the nutritional needs of a healthy full-term baby. (For the needs of premature or sick babies taking formula, please refer to Chapter 8).

There are two main types of protein found in milk: whey and casein. Human milk in the early weeks contains about a 60:40 ratio of whey to casein, whereas cow's milk is closer to 20:80, with a much higher protein content overall. First infant milk is modified so that the ratio is 60:40, like human milk, but the overall protein content remains higher. The NHS recommends using a whey-based milk based on cow's or goat's milk.[8]

Confusingly, there are some products that will be labelled 'suitable from birth' that actually aren't. These products make claims like 'easier to digest' or that they will promote sleep, which are not substantiated by any evidence, and contain ingredients like glucose and corn syrup which can be harmful to babies. The main products that this applies to are *comfort milk* and *hungry baby milk*.

Hungry baby milk has a whey:casein ratio of 20:80, which is why it takes longer for the baby to digest it. This may put a strain on immature digestive systems, and lead to excessive weight gain because of the high levels of protein.

Comfort milk usually contains protein that has been broken down (partially hydrolysed), and is marketed as being easier to digest and sometimes as preventing allergies. There is no clinical evidence that either of these claims is true.

Not generally suitable from birth

There are a number of other products out there which parents may consider using in specific circumstances, although there is often no evidence that these different milks offer any health benefits over whey-based first infant milk.

Lactose-free formula is available for babies who have lactose intolerance. Lactose is a sugar found naturally in milk, and is digested by an enzyme called lactase. Most babies are born with enough lactase to digest milk, and sometimes the amount of lactase produced decreases as the person ages and they start to eat a more diverse diet. In some cases, a baby has insufficient lactase, or no lactase at all, and under medical supervision, can be provided with lactose-free formula. This is not suitable for healthy babies, for whom lactose has a role in the digestive system.

Anti-reflux milk should again only be used under medical supervision. Most babies are sick a lot, and many of the symptoms of reflux are also signs either of a breastfeeding issue (which may well have a breastfeeding solution) or a bottle-feeding approach that overwhelms the baby (see Chapter 5 for suggestions about this). However, if the baby is clearly unwell, and in particular if they are not gaining weight, and issues with breastfeeding or bottle-feeding have been explored with appropriate specialists, then anti-reflux milk might be considered. This type of milk contains a thickener, and must be made up with water at a lower temperature than the NHS guidelines recommend (see 'Preparing it correctly' below).

Follow-on milk, growing-up milk, and *toddler milk* are not suitable for babies under six months because of the whey:protein ratio, and have no nutritional benefits over first infant milk for babies over six months. From the age of one year, babies can have unmodified cow or goat milk.

Soya-based formula is not recommended for babies under six months without medical supervision, and is not protective against allergies. In fact some babies may be more at risk of allergies using this milk, and in addition there is a potentially harmful effect on future fertility owing to phyto-oestrogens in soya-protein-based milk, and a higher risk of dental decay due to the presence of the sugar maltodextrin.

There are very few *vegetarian formula milks*, as many contain fish oils or rennet. The FAQ on infantmilkinfo.org has up-to-date information on this. And there are no *vegan formula milks* as all formula contains Vitamin D from animal sources.

Some *Halal formula* is available; check infantmilkinfo.org for up-to-date information.

There is no evidence that *organic formula milk*[9] offers any nutritional or health benefits, and indeed if it did then this would be a requirement of all formula milk. There is some evidence that organic milk production is better for the environment as a whole, though not necessarily in terms of animal welfare.

Preparing it correctly

This is *essential*, because powdered formula is not sterile, and milk offers a fertile growth environment for bacteria, including dangerous food poisoning bacteria such as *E.coli* and *Salmonella*. Factories where formula is prepared are not sterile, and the powder is not heat treated after production because this would affect its nutritional content. Your parents or grandparents may well have made up several bottles at once and used them over the course of the day and night, but current guidelines recommend very strongly that you make up feeds as you go, to reduce the risk of the baby ingesting these harmful bacteria. It can be hard to go against what your own parents remember doing, but science has advanced and we now know much more about the potential harms of unsafe milk preparation.

Making it up

Guidelines from the NHS, UNICEF and Start4Life all offer a 14-point step-by-step approach, which is what I am using here.

Ensure all equipment is clean and sterilised (see Chapter 5)

1. Boil up to one litre of *tap water*.
   Do not use softened water or water that has already been boiled. Bottled water usually has high sodium and sulphate levels, so check these. Sodium (Na) should be less than 200mg per litre, and sulphate (SO_4) less than 250mg per litre.

2. Leave the water to cool in the kettle for *no more than 30 minutes*, so that it remains *above 70°C*. This is so that the water is hot enough to sterilise the powder and kill bacteria. You do not need to wait the full 30 minutes, but can add the water to the powder immediately. This will ensure it is definitely hot enough, and saves time.

3. Clean and disinfect the surfaces you are going to use.

4. Wash your hands.

5. If you use a cold-water sterilising solution, shake off excess solution, or rinse bottle and teat using boiled water.

6. Stand the bottle on a clean surface.

7. Keep the teat and cap in the steriliser or the steriliser lid, so that they don't contact non-sterile surfaces.

8. Check the instructions on the packet, and add the exact amount of boiled water to the bottle. Double check the amount before adding powder.

9. Measure the powder using the scoop provided, which should be loosely filled and not packed down. Level it off with the leveller provided or a clean dry knife. Ensure you use the exact quantity stated on the packet.

10. Handling by the edges, place the teat on top of the bottle, and screw the retaining ring into place.
11. Put the cap on the bottle and shake gently until the powder has dissolved.
12. Cool the formula so that it is a safe temperature to drink, by holding it under a running cold tap.
13. Test the temperature by dropping a little formula on to the inside of your wrist. If it is body temperature, this will feel neither hot nor cold, and this will be suitable for your baby.
14. If there is any formula left when the baby is finished (see 'paced bottle feeding' in Chapter 5), you must throw this away.

Important things to note:

- It is important to make up the formula according to the packet instructions, because if the mixture is too strong or too weak, your baby will not be getting the right balance of nutrients. Formula that is too strong can cause dehydration and constipation. Always use the scoop provided with the pack you are using, as sizes and quantities may change from batch to batch.
- Never add anything else (e.g. cereal) to the bottle, as this can be a choking hazard.
- Do not warm formula in the microwave, as this heats the milk unevenly and can scald your baby.
- Formula that has been made up but not used, or ready-made formula that has been opened but not used, should be discarded once it has been at room temperature for two hours.

Formula preparation machines

These machines save some preparation time, but they are costly, and importantly, may not allow the user to follow the safe preparation guidelines: specifically, the amount of hot water mixed with the powder is not enough for it to stay hot for long enough to kill any bacteria.

Ready-to-feed liquid formula

Formula that is ready-made and comes in cartons or bottles is sterile until the carton or bottle is opened. This can be quick and convenient, particularly when out and about; and may also reduce the risk of vulnerable babies coming into contact with harmful bacteria. It is, however, significantly more expensive. Remember that the composition is basically the same as powdered formula, so you might consider using liquid occasionally but mostly rely on the powder.

Once opened, decant a small quantity into a feeding bottle. You can always add more, but you will need to throw away anything that the baby doesn't take from the bottle.

You may warm the milk, following the instructions on the packet; or you may find that your baby is happy to take it at room temperature, or even (when they are a little older) cold from the fridge.

If there is any milk left in the original container, seal this or turn the carton corner down and store it in the back of the fridge (where it is coldest) for up to 24 hours.

'I used pre-made formula. This suited me perfectly because I could use it as and when I wanted to/needed to. I didn't have to do any preparation, just threw some [ready-made] 200ml bottles in my bag and I was prepared for anything. This actually saved my sanity, I felt less guilty because it felt like a "backup" rather than

a hard choice between breast and formula. I felt less anxiety about breastfeeding out and about knowing I had my backup.' Ali

Formula tablets

Currently one brand offers a tablet, equivalent to a pre-measured scoop of powder. The manufacturer claims that this reduces mess and wastage, but it does create packaging waste, and the product is still not sterile. It is not clear whether hot water penetrates the tablet quickly enough to decontaminate it, and it is not recommended to use them with preparation machines for that reason.

Making up formula outside the home

If you need to make up formula when you are away from home, and will not have access to a kettle in order to follow the steps described, then you will need to prepare the following in advance:

- a sterilised bottle, sealed with the cap;
- pre-measured powder in a clean, lidded container; and
- boiled water in a vacuum flask.

A sealed vacuum flask should keep the water hot enough for several hours (check the manufacturer's information). Make the feed when needed, remembering to cool it before offering it to the baby.

If you absolutely must make up the feed before you go out, follow the step-by-step instructions, and then cool it for at least one hour in the back of the fridge, before taking it with you in a cool bag. Use it within four hours.

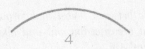

What do parents need to know about expressing breastmilk?

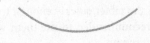

Expressing breastmilk means getting milk out of the breast without the help of a baby, by using a breast pump or your hands to gently extract it. This can happen for a whole range of different reasons. In this chapter we will look at what those reasons are, and how you might go about it. There are very few books with comprehensive information about expressing, but the NHS and all the main breastfeeding charities have good information on their websites. There are books that support expressing in specific situations, such as when the mother is trying to increase her own milk supply, or when caring for a premature baby.

> 'I pumped for some of his top-ups but was unable, to start with, to produce enough, so we had to use formula (pretty much from day 1). Eventually the amount I was pumping increased, and we ditched the formula, then he got strong enough to feed directly himself, and we ditched the bottles.' Hilary

Oxytocin

Back in Chapter 2, we looked at the hormones that have a role in breastfeeding, and you may (if not too sleep-deprived) remember that oxytocin helps breastmilk to flow. Oxytocin is a shy hormone, which reacts badly to stress and discomfort, so when expressing, my best suggestion is to do everything you can to do it somewhere you feel comfortable, safe and private, and to rope in your supporters to help you with this.

You may have noticed how cute babies generally are, with their big eyes and button noses and amazing baby smell. All of this cuteness is enough to release oxytocin in anyone, but especially (in most cases) their mother. Sometimes she doesn't even need the baby nearby, but may find that a picture of the baby or a piece of their clothing stimulates oxytocin. All of this is helpful for the flow of milk. If you've ever had the opportunity to examine a breast pump, on the other hand, you may have noticed their utter lack of cuteness or oxytocin-inducing properties. They have, in fact, been known to cause feelings of stress with a single glance. It is for this reason that some mothers find it difficult to express milk: it will usually flow more readily for a baby, or in conditions of elevated oxytocin. So if some well-meaning advisor suggests to you that you express milk in order to 'see how much you've got', do remember that the quantity you can get out with a pump is unlikely to be a reliable indication of the amount of milk you can produce in optimal circumstances. Perhaps your well-meaning advisor could be better employed trying to help you to optimise those circumstances.

The production of breastmilk relies on more than just removing milk from the breast, though this is key. Expressing instead of breastfeeding will generally not be as good at establishing a milk supply as effective direct breastfeeding. Expressing as well as breastfeeding will usually increase the supply.

Why do people express breastmilk?

There are two very broad categories here:

1. Because you need to.
2. Because you want to.

Some situations might fit into both categories. Let's try and break them down a bit further.

Situations where you might feel like you have to express milk

To establish a milk supply, where the newborn baby is not able to breastfeed directly, and therefore also to have some colostrum or breastmilk for the baby. If your baby is not breastfeeding at all, then the ideal strategy would be to express between 8 and 10 times over 24 hours, including at least once in the night. This is because frequent stimulation of the breasts works to increase prolactin and therefore milk production, and there are higher levels of prolactin in the mother's bloodstream at night (and in fact this is stimulated by broken sleep, as some sort of rather shoddy compensation for the lack of rest). However, and I cannot emphasise enough how important this is: ANY amount of expressing that you can manage is helpful, both for your milk supply and to provide some breastmilk for your baby. If it is possible to have skin-to-skin time with your baby, this will be helpful in lots of ways, including to stimulate the release of both prolactin and oxytocin.

> 'I struggled to pump anything and also giving one bottle of formula a day seemed the easiest way to do it, given all other feeds were from the breast.' Marie

It may also be useful, if you are in this situation, to read Chapter 8 on mixed feeding premature or sick babies.

This situation might also arise where *the baby does not latch on, or feeding is extremely painful.* That is, mother and baby are not separated, but the breastfeeding is not quite happening, so the mother is expressing to establish the milk supply, while also seeking high-quality breastfeeding support from the infant feeding team, a breastfeeding counsellor, or a lactation consultant.

To maintain the milk supply, when direct breastfeeding is interrupted. For example, if the mother is taking medication that genuinely* means she can't breastfeed, or if mother and baby are to be separated for any other reason, whether this is a hen party or a work trip or a hospital procedure, or anything else that might come up for you. The other reason why you might express milk in this situation is to manage engorgement and reduce the risk of mastitis (see below).

In this case, you can express roughly at the time when your baby would usually feed, or at any time when the breasts become uncomfortably full. You may find that even with a bit of expressing going on, your supply still dips a bit. When it is possible for the baby to return to the breast, they may feed more intensively than usual, to build it back up again.

> 'I was worried about sleep deprivation and wanted my baby to be okay with a bottle so I could be free to go out for a day (I have a hen do coming up).' Stephanie

To increase milk supply, because the more milk is removed from the breast, the more milk is produced. Milk removal

---

* Most medications are compatible or manageable with breastfeeding. If you've been told that breastfeeding needs to stop, either temporarily or permanently, because of medication that you need to take, do please seek a second opinion from a breastfeeding specialist such as breastfeeding-and-medication.co.uk

stimulates prolactin, and reduces the amount of feedback inhibitor of lactation (FIL) present, and therefore milk production increases. To optimise this, frequent, short expressing sessions are more helpful than one or two long sessions would be. Some women try 'power pumping', which is to express for just a few minutes after each feed. Others find 'cluster pumping', mimicking a baby's very frequent feeds over a shorter time period, to be helpful. Different sources will define these terms differently, which can be confusing; see which one works for you, and don't worry about what it's called.

> 'We were readmitted to hospital [on] day 5 for weight loss (14% – she was 11lb at birth) so needed a formula top-up alongside breastfeeding and expressed top-up every 3 hours. My husband was absolutely vital in those first days and weeks – after the initial breast feed, he would do the bottle-feeding (breastmilk then formula) so I could move onto pumping. He would also do the sterilising/running bottles to and from the fridge etc.' Violet

To relieve engorgement, and prevent or resolve mastitis. Engorgement (fullness) occurs when the milk remains in the breast a little longer than usual, causing inflammation of the breast tissue. The milk is not affected by this, and so can be given to the baby. However, when the breasts are engorged, babies can sometimes struggle to latch well, because the surface of the breast is stretched firmer and flatter than usual. Briefly expressing (ideally by hand, as this can be more gentle), to remove some milk, should soften the breast and make it easier for the baby to latch on. You may then want to store the milk rather than using it immediately, so that the baby takes what they need directly from the breast. This then should help the supply to equalise against the baby's need, and give the baby practice to refine their breastfeeding skills.

When engorgement is not relieved, either by feeding the baby or expressing, it can escalate to mastitis, which is uncomfortable fullness, along with flu-like symptoms such as fever, headache and tiredness. It is not recommended to do lots of expressing to resolve mastitis. The current protocol for treating mastitis is well explained by Sarah Oakley here: sarahoakleylactation. co.uk/wp-content/uploads/2021/03/mastitis.pdf. A warm bath or shower, cold compresses to reduce the inflammation, hot compresses to encourage the flow of milk, and over-the-counter anti-inflammatories (if it is safe for the mother to use these) can also help. If the symptoms of mastitis do not resolve within about 24 hours, the GP may be able to prescribe antibiotics. Most antibiotics are compatible with breastfeeding, and – again – this is a condition of the breast tissue that does not affect the milk itself, and so the milk should be safe for the baby. If you take antibiotics, it is still important to remove the milk from the breast as well.

Situations where you might want to express breastmilk

So that someone else can feed the baby, whether this is a regular thing or a one-off situation.

> *'I planned ideally, breastfeeding and bottle-feeding of expressed milk (to include the father). We wanted to avoid formula.'* Agi

For the *occasional separation* such as a hen party, a hair appointment, or a Keeping In Touch day at work, where you have arranged for someone else to care for the baby (their other parent, for example, or a childminder), you may wish to express breastmilk for the baby's feeds during the time you are apart. It is likely to be a good idea to start building your stash in advance, rather than hope to express the whole amount needed the day before you need it (we will come on to handling and storage shortly). Try frequent short expressing sessions, whenever it is convenient to do so, and store the milk in small quantities, so that it is not wasted if the baby doesn't take all of it. As mentioned above, you may also need to express during the time you are apart, to relieve engorgement and also to maintain your milk supply if it is a longer separation.

In the event of a *planned, regular separation*, for example when you go back to work, do talk to your employer about arrangements for you to express. The Health and Safety Executive (HSE) guidance recommends that employers provide access to a private room where you can breastfeed or express; somewhere suitable to store expressed milk while you are at work; and facilities to wash, sterilise, and store equipment. You have no legal right to paid breastfeeding breaks, but many employers do offer these.[1]

Often when a mother goes back to work after breastfeeding is well-established, her supply can handle some disruptions during the day, and the baby may well do more of their breastfeeding during the evenings/nights or on days when the mother is not at work. Do consider what support you may need to cope with this.

It is very common for new parents to plan *to express so that both parents can feed the baby,* to give the mother the opportunity to get some sleep, and so that her partner can spend time with the baby, which we discussed in Chapter 1. Unfortunately, while they can share the feeding, mothers cannot share the chore of expressing. This is what gives rise to the idea that it's not a good idea to express in the first few weeks if you don't have to: the newborn period can be a busy, busy time, and finding space in your day to express milk may not feel like your top priority.

However, this is not a non-negotiable rule; if you feel like you can fit it in, by all means have a go.

'I wish I had known when to pump, and that I didn't have to wait until six weeks.' Charlotte

There are some things to consider, if this is the plan. Firstly, as mentioned, when to express. There is no evidence that expressing at one time of the day will be any easier than any other time, but mothers often feel that there is a surplus of milk available in the morning, following those high night-time levels of prolactin.

Next you need to think about how to allocate a feeding time to the non-breastfeeding parent. In the early days (and often later) it is unlikely that a healthy, full-term breastfeeding baby will have set feeding times. So it may be easier to allocate a 'window' – for example, if the baby wakes between 10pm and midnight, this could be an opportunity for your partner to feed them. Would this work better for your family than to do the bottle-feed in the small hours of the morning? One side-effect of prolactin is hypervigilance, meaning that the breastfeeding parent will tend to find it easier to wake from sleep and respond to the baby, than the parent who isn't breastfeeding.

If the baby has been feeding frequently round the clock, then when you insert a bottle-feed into this picture, the mother may still need to express milk to prevent engorgement. This means she is not necessarily getting any extra rest in this scenario, and is another reason why it can work better after a few weeks than in the early days. When breastfeeding is more established, it is easier to manage the milk supply against the baby's need. This means that, while the mother may need to express during the bottle-feeding 'window' the first few nights, she can express a little less each night until this is no longer needed. This of course implies that she will need to find another time of the day to express, for breastmilk to be available for the bottle-feed.

I can see that the last few paragraphs may make this whole exercise sound daunting and almost not worth the effort. It does work very well for some families, while others have to experiment a lot until they find a routine that works for them. If you try it and find that it hasn't made things easier for you after all, don't be afraid to go back to what you were doing, give yourself a little time, and then try again. Things change all the time when you have a new baby, and what doesn't work at two weeks may work like a dream at two months. Give yourself a break.

To mix up purees or add to solid food. See Amy Brown's *Why Starting Solids Matters* for more on this.

To donate breastmilk to a milk bank. The UK has about 14 milk banks where donated milk is available, usually for sick and premature babies in the hospital where the milk bank is based. We will come back to this in Chapter 8 on mixed feeding your sick or premature baby.

When the mother/chestfeeding parent does not want to breastfeed directly, whether this is occasional (for example, to help with anxiety about breastfeeding outside the home) or a more regular thing, such as when someone has trauma or dysphoria about this part of their body, a history of sexual abuse, or in a culture where breastfeeding cannot be seen by men.

'I exclusively pumped all the breastmilk I fed rather than breastfeeding, [and] produced about 80% of all the milk for the first five months then switched to all formula after that.' Louise

A word about growth spurts

There is a theory that babies have sudden periods of rapid growth, which fall at particular times. However, every internet parenting forum will show you countless examples of these 'growth spurts' that have popped up either a bit early or a bit late, which suggests to me that they occur randomly. What we can say is that some days the baby will feed a bit more intensively, and that this can be a completely normal way for them to meet their needs for extra comfort, food or security as they arise. It often happens after they've had their vaccinations, or following a really busy sociable day when they've been passed around every member of their extended family twice and not had much time in the safe haven of their mother's arms (and therefore not much opportunity to breastfeed). If a baby is a bit under the weather, or the mother's milk supply has dipped perhaps because of a brief separation, or indeed during one of these utterly random and unpredictable growth spurts, the baby may feed more to build up the supply, so that it continues to meet their needs. This is how it works: the more milk the baby removes, the more the mother's body makes.

Some popular parenting books recommend expressing in advance, in order to keep up with growth spurts. In fact this can make things much more complicated, as it requires time to be spent expressing before it is needed, and then prevents the milk supply from building in line with the baby's needs, by supplementing breastfeeds with the stash of expressed milk.

Other ways to manage these periods of intensive feeding are to seek support from those around you, and foster their understanding that you might not get much else done if the baby is feeding more than usual. This is a good opportunity to enjoy an audiobook or box set, and remember that your baby isn't going to be this tiny and needy forever, and that they are redeemingly cute. If you are worried that something doesn't feel quite right, do seek good-quality breastfeeding support, because as your baby grows and gets heavier, their latch may change, which could contribute to longer or more frequent feeding.

> 'Pumping gives you even more freedom and flexibility but you need a lot of support to make it work.' Louise

How to express breastmilk

Different methods of expressing will suit different situations. If you are separated from your baby, and/or attempting to express enough to meet all or the majority of their needs, then some sort of fairly heavy-duty electric pump will probably be useful. If you are just expressing now and then to relieve engorgement, or for someone else to give an occasional bottle, then a manual pump will probably be adequate. And women's bodies respond differently to different pumps. Since it is possible to acquire a pump reasonably quickly, it may be worth waiting to see what you need it for, before you invest.

With any pump, it is important that the 'flange', or funnel, fits comfortably over the nipple, so that it does not hurt; different sizes are sometimes available, especially for the larger rental pumps – speak to the person you are hiring from to find out more. Expressing milk should be comfortable; if it hurts, then definitely look at the flange size or consider using something to lubricate the flange. Note that your breasts might not be exactly the same size, and you may need different flanges for left and right.

Different types of pump

Expressing by hand doesn't require a pump at all. This is

most commonly suggested for antenatal or early postnatal expressing of colostrum, but it can be done at any time. This lends itself well to gently relieving engorgement by hand-expressing in the bath or shower, or at any time when you don't have access to a pump. There are numerous videos on YouTube and Instagram demonstrating how to do this.

Collecting 'drip milk' using a breast shell or a one-piece silicone breast pump. These devices collect the milk that leaks from the breast not currently feeding. You can also hand express into the silicone breast pump. Not everyone leaks copiously, but if this is you, it can save you some time. These items are cheap to buy, easy to clean, and don't take up a lot of space. The silicone breast pump creates a small amount of suction, so can collect a little more than only the milk that drips, and may actively but slightly increase the milk supply. Drip milk tends to be slightly lower in fat than normal expressed breastmilk, so would not be suitable to make up the majority of a baby's diet, but it can supplement breastfeeding or formula.

A manual breastpump is, unsurprisingly, one that you operate by hand. This means you can control the strength and speed of suction, making it good for relieving engorgement and other situations where gentleness is key. If expressing isn't going to be a huge part of your life, this pump will probably meet your needs nicely. There is a wide range available, all working on similar principles, but some are just better made than others. Some brands provide a microwave steriliser, bottles and feeding cups in a kit with the pump. Manual pumps are cheaper than electric pumps, and good when you don't have access to a power supply.

Electric breastpumps come in single and double, i.e. to be used on one breast at a time, or simultaneously on both, which is particularly good if you need to build up a milk supply, or if you find yourself having to produce a lot of expressed milk for your baby. It's overkill for occasional expressing; these things are expensive and usually bulky, with complicated parts that you do or don't need to sterilise – do check the instructions that come with them, and bear in mind that you can usually get spares from the manufacturer.

Hospital-grade electric pumps are usually double, with a large heavy unit, and are either loaned by the hospital, for example where a baby is in the Neonatal Unit, or can be rented directly from the manufacturer. In some areas local charities or community centres can also rent them out. Rental is expensive in the long term, but if you only need it for a week or two, then it is cheaper than buying an electric pump.

Wearable breast pumps are also available from a number of different manufacturers. These are like a soft cup that sits in the bra, so that the mother can go about her day without having to allocate time for expressing. This works really well for people who need to be distracted for the pumping to work, and not so well for people who find they need to focus on it. You may have a feel for how this would apply to you. These devices are high tech, and not cheap.

You will find numerous articles online telling you which is the best pump, but it's very hard to know how your body will respond. I found the electric pump very useful in the early weeks when I was building a supply, but later when I went back to work, and was only expressing once a day, the manual pump was absolutely adequate, and light and easy to carry into the office with me.

Some suggestions to optimise expressing

Keep in mind these three main principles:

1. Any amount that you produce is an achievement

2.   Oxytocin helps milk to flow
3.   Milk removal creates milk production

Since oxytocin helps, there are a few things you can do, or ask someone supporting you to do, to increase your levels of this hormone. Look at your environment and think about how to make it more relaxing, whether that's simply by closing the door, evicting the visitors, and adding cushions or music or food or all three. If it's possible to have your baby close or even skin-to-skin, that's going to help. If it isn't possible, a picture of them or a piece of clothing could also work.

Perhaps it's easier said than done, but allow time. Nobody is going to be able to tell you how long it will take to express a certain amount of milk, so if you're building up a stash for someone else to feed, give yourself a good run-up.

Depending on how much you can control the action of the pump, start with fast cycles and low suction. After a few minutes you will notice drips of milk. As this begins to increase, turn the cycles down, and the suction up, mimicking what the baby would do if they were feeding directly. Do not turn it up so high that it hurts.

Do not panic if you don't get much the first time, especially if it's very early in the life of your baby. Remember that first principle: any amount that you produce is an achievement.

Even if your baby is not directly breastfeeding, spending time cuddling them skin-to-skin, and allowing them to nuzzle at the breast, will stimulate the milk production hormones, as well as give you some pleasant bonding time.

Frequent short expressing sessions will generally get a better yield than one long one. You do not have to sterilise your equipment in between expressing sessions on the same day: you can put it all in the fridge, and sterilise once in 24 hours. Milk can be mixed for storage, as long as a new batch is cooled first before adding to the earlier milk, and dated from the first batch produced.

The amount you can get will vary from session to session. This is normal.

If you are using a single pump, frequent switching usually helps to increase the yield. Start with five minutes on each side, then do four minutes on each side, then three, then two, then one. Then stop – that's plenty.

Some mothers find it helpful to cover the collection bottle (a baby sock fits nicely) so that they can't see how much is coming out. This may alleviate pressure to produce lots of milk.

Remember that third principle: milk removal creates milk production. So if you have just pumped, and your baby needs to feed, this is okay – the body responds to the baby by making milk. Equally, immediately following a feed could be a good time to pump, as there is usually a lot of oxytocin in the system at this point. The breast is never completely empty, but when it is emptier, milk production steps up.

If you're thinking about starting to express to allow someone to share feeding, look at your day. Is there an obvious time when you can fit it in? If not, could you wait until there is? If expressing feels like it is going to add to your burden, rather than alleviate it, perhaps this isn't the right time.

If you are expressing to relieve engorgement, then just express enough to make the breast softer and more comfortable, and if possible then revert to breastfeeding directly. This is also a good strategy if you are stopping breastfeeding, and gradually reducing your supply.

Storage and handling of expressed breastmilk

There is a difference between the *optimal* amount of time that breastmilk can be stored, and the *safe* amount of time. I'm going to share with you the NHS[2] guidance, but obviously if it can be stored for shorter periods, so much the better. During storage, some nutrients will degrade; however, unless your baby is only having breastmilk that has been stored for long periods, it is still going to provide nutritious food.

Chill the milk as quickly as possible. Use a sterilised container or special breastmilk storage bag, and store it in small quantities to prevent waste.

At room temperature, the milk can be stored for 6–8 hours. This means that if you express it and know you will be using it in a few hours' time, there is no need to refrigerate, and therefore no need to heat it.

In a typical domestic fridge, it will keep for up to eight days. Do check that your fridge temperature is 4°C or less. If it isn't, then use the milk within three days. Store it at the back of the fridge, where it is coldest, in a container that can be labelled with the date. Milk that has been refrigerated can be carried in a cool bag with an ice pack for 24 hours.

In the ice compartment of a fridge, it will keep safely for two weeks.

In a freezer, which should be below -18°C, you can store breastmilk for up to six months.

Defrost the milk overnight in the fridge if possible, or by immersing the container in warm water. Use immediately and throw away any that the baby does not drink within an hour.

Warm the milk, if necessary, by immersing the container in warm water. Babies will often accept milk at room temperature, and slightly older babies may take it at fridge temperature.

5

What do parents need to know about using bottles and other feeding devices?

Feeding your baby, no matter what type of milk you are using, is about nurturing as well as nourishment. So while there are some important facts I can share with you about different types of bottles and so on, the most important thing to remind you of is *responsive feeding*. In Chapter 2, we looked at responding to your baby's feeding cues, and this is just as applicable when the baby is having a bottle as when they are breastfeeding.

Paced bottle-feeding

Parents often express anxiety about doing harm by giving a bottle. They may feel that they can more easily overfeed with a bottle, or that using a bottle will cause their baby to lose the ability to breastfeed. Given that the bottle is often used when the baby is already struggling to breastfeed, it won't help them to learn or refine their breastfeeding skills, but it will help them to get the milk they need, and this can be done alongside getting skilled breastfeeding support.

Current guidance talks about paced bottle-feeding, which

is thought to help both with the worry about overfeeding, in that it allows the baby to control how much they take and how fast they take it, and with enabling the baby to manage both of these different skills without losing one or the other.

You may have seen babies being given a bottle in a position where they are lying almost on their back, and the bottle pours milk down from above. As the bottle teat touches at the back of the baby's palate, where a nipple would be if the baby was at the breast, it elicits the baby's sucking action. This in turn draws milk from the bottle, which the baby must swallow. It is difficult for the baby to control the flow of milk, as it is coming from above.

It is now recommended that the baby is positioned much more upright, tucked in close to the parent just as they would be at the breast. The parent can have good eye contact and interact with the baby, as well as monitor for signs that the baby needs a break. The bottle is then level with the baby, and at a more horizontal angle, so that milk doesn't pour from the teat. Touch the teat to the baby's lips and let them latch on, as they would at the breast. Allow the baby frequent breaks, and do not encourage the baby to continue feeding after they have stopped. Usually they will turn their head away or close their mouth when they have had enough: trust your baby to regulate their intake of food, as this is a skill that is useful in later life.

Some parents will choose to swap the baby to the opposite side part-way through a bottle feed, to give them a different visual stimulus. This is entirely up to you. Remember you need to discard any unused milk within an hour.

This video from lactation consultant Emma Pickett shows paced bottle feeding: www.emmapickettbreastfeedingsupport. com/twitter-and-blog/giving-a-breastfed-baby-their-first-bottle

Nipple confusion

There is a deeply entrenched belief that giving a baby a bottle will cause them to 'forget' the reflexes that enable them to breastfeed. There is little evidence for this.[1]

> *'I didn't want to get my baby into the habit of just not trying at the breast, because he knows a bottle of milk will show up if he doesn't latch on.'* Sindy

So let's clear this up. Babies are born with reflexes that help them to breastfeed, and you will notice your baby showing you these when they want to feed: rooting or turning the head, gaping the mouth and smacking the lips, and getting increasingly fidgety with their arms and legs. If the baby is placed so that they can use these reflexes (e.g. well supported on their mother's body, with their head near to the breast), they can often position themselves in order to get a good latch. As long as the mother is able to continue supporting the baby in this position, the baby should then latch on and feed. If the baby is struggling to do this, the chances are that adjusting the baby's position, or seeking some specialist breastfeeding support, will help.

Your newborn baby is incapable of remembering that an object exists if they cannot see it. This ability (called 'object permanence'[2]) develops at around eight months of age. Nor does your newborn baby have the mental capacity to plan, or any concept of cause and effect. This means that they cannot, on being put to the breast, think to themselves, 'Ah, if I just don't bother with this boring old latching on business, she'll give me a nice easy bottle of milk to drink'. Your baby's every instinct is to breastfeed, and they will do the very best they can with what they've got. If they can't latch on, it's because they can't, not because they won't, or they're lazy, or they're naughty. Again, you can reach out for some breastfeeding support to try to help them.

It is often the case that, in a situation where the baby is struggling to latch on for any reason, they are offered milk in a bottle. While the bottle won't give them the opportunity to refine and practice their breastfeeding skills, it's not going to teach them that they don't have to bother, and it's not going to cause those reflexes to vanish. Regularly using a bottle might, however, have an impact on the mother's milk supply, which could result in the baby being less satisfied or comfortable at the breast. This too is worth exploring with a breastfeeding counsellor or lactation consultant.

So using a bottle does not, in itself, undermine a baby's ability to breastfeed. But it can happen in a situation where the baby's ability to breastfeed is already compromised, and it can affect the availability of milk at the breast. Nonetheless, parents sometimes get warned ominously about the dire consequences of using a bottle, or blame themselves for a situation that quite possibly could not have been avoided.

Alternatives to the bottle

In some situations, it is appropriate to use something other than a bottle to feed your baby. You should be able to ask your midwife to support you with this at home or on the postnatal ward, as needed. When using any of these methods, hold your baby close and securely, both for their wellbeing, and to reduce wastage and mess from spilt milk.

Cup feeding

Milk is put in a special feeding cup (rather like the lid of a feeding bottle in size and shape), and this is tilted towards the baby's mouth. The baby laps it like a kitten. It can be messy; you may want to drape the baby and surrounding adult with muslin cloths. The advantages of this over any of the methods using tubing are that less fat is lost than on the sides of the tube, and it's easier to clean and sterilise a cup.

Sometimes parents choose to do this because they are worried that introducing a bottle will have a greater impact on the baby's ability to breastfeed, but there is no evidence that this is the case, and the paced feeding method described above may be an alternative to consider.

Finger feeding

This is where the milk is put in a small container that can be held in the hand, with a thin tube taped to the finger. The finger is then inserted into the baby's mouth for them to suck on. This is not going to be suitable for large volumes, but may work in the short term for a newborn or premature baby.

Spoon feeding

Using a spoon to give milk can work, but again it is not really suitable for large volumes. As with the cup, you would let the baby lap the milk, rather than insert the spoon into their mouth.

Syringes

These are usually used for small amounts of colostrum, and you may have been given 1ml syringes before the birth, in order to collect some colostrum. You can get syringes with larger capacity, up to 10ml. Place the syringe into the side of the baby's cheek alongside a clean finger, so that you can feel when the baby sucks, and depress the syringe only when they are sucking.

All of the above are for consideration if your baby cannot latch on at the breast, but can swallow. Please do talk to a midwife or lactation consultant for support with how to obtain and use the equipment.

Supplementary nursing systems

A supplementary nursing system (SNS) or breastfeeding supplementer is usually used where the baby can latch on, but the mother's milk supply is compromised or insufficient for the baby to get all of their milk directly from the breast. This can be useful in cases of induced lactation, for example adoptive mothers, lesbian mothers who did not give birth, or in cases where a transgender parent wants to feed at the breast. Depending on the amount of milk the parent is producing, the baby may also need additional feeds from a bottle or other feeding method.

The SNS consists of a container of milk, and one or two thin tubes. The container is suspended around the neck, and the tubes, which lead from the container, are taped at the nipple. The baby can then latch on at the breast and feed, getting milk from both the breast and the container. This means that there is some stimulation to the milk-producing hormone prolactin, and the baby is able to continue refining their breastfeeding skills.

Choosing bottles

There is no evidence that any make or style of bottle is better than any other make or style of bottle, including those making claims of 'colic relief' or 'being more like a breast'. It is immaterial how much a bottle looks like a breast, and also a bit bonkers – bottles look nothing like breasts, and don't act like them either!

Therefore the question of which bottle is easily answered: choose one that is inexpensive and easy to clean, with clear calibrations on the side. You can check how well the bottle is calibrated by weighing the water on a set of digital scales: 1fl oz weighs 1oz, and 1ml weighs 1g (of water).

Teats

The teat needs to fit the bottle properly, so you may be tied to buying teats from the same manufacturer as the bottle. Most ranges will offer different flow rates: 'slow', 'medium' or 'fast' teats. Start with slow, as this will be easier for the baby to manage. There is no competitive element here: move on to a faster teat if you think your baby needs it, but do not feel under pressure to make your baby feed more quickly.

Teats are available in silicone or latex. Latex is usually a bit softer, but some people avoid it because of allergies. Manufacturers recommend that you replace the teats roughly every two months.

Cleaning and sterilising

You need to clean *and* sterilise anything that comes into contact with formula milk, so bottles and teats. The NHS recommends continuing to sterilise feeding equipment for the first 12 months. If you wish to, you can buy special brushes for cleaning bottles and teats. Breast pumps and bottles used with expressed breastmilk can be thoroughly cleaned, but do not have to be sterilised before each use. Only sterilise the parts of the pump that come into contact with milk, i.e. not the tubing that creates the pump's suction.

You have various options to choose from, based on what will work best in your own circumstances.

Boiling

This is a low-tech option, but is time-consuming because you probably need to keep an eye on the pan, and it will gradually damage the bottles and teats. Bring the water to the boil, then put the equipment into the water and boil it for 10 minutes. Ideally take the bottles out of the water just before you need them. If this isn't practical, put them together with the lid on to keep the inside of the bottle sterile.

Cold-water sterilising

Sterilising solution is available as tablets or fluid, which you would dilute in a large lidded container. Equipment needs to be in the liquid for at least 15 minutes (check the instructions in case this is different), but will remain sterile as long as it is in there. Change the solution every 24 hours. There is no need to rinse, but shake off any excess liquid before using.

Steam sterilising

This can be done in a microwave, using either a plastic steriliser unit (these are sometimes supplied with breast pumps) or multi-use disposable sterilising bags. Or you can invest in a steam steriliser, which will usually be a bit bigger and more expensive. As with boiling, it will take around 10 minutes to sterilise your equipment, but check the manufacturer's instructions for your steriliser. The instructions will also tell you how long items will remain sterile if left inside the container.

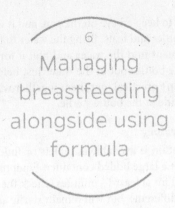

6

Managing breastfeeding alongside using formula

For mixed feeding to work, the mother or chestfeeding parent needs to maintain a supply of breastmilk to meet the needs of their baby alongside the expressed breastmilk or formula. How this happens will depend on the circumstances and the long-term plan. I will try to break it down into some broad themes, and hope that you can find something here that applies to you and is useful. We will look here at using formula milk alongside breastfeeding, and managing the milk supply to increase or decrease it according to your preference and longer-term plan. You may wish to move towards less breastfeeding, in which case there are some things to consider for this to happen safely.

Using formula milk alongside breastfeeding is, as we said at the beginning of the book, far and away the most common way to feed a baby under six months old in the UK. It happens in broadly three different ways: intentionally, from the start; intentionally after a few weeks; and unplanned when there are issues with breastfeeding.

'I always planned exclusive breastfeeding with one bottle of formula before bed'. Grace

'I decided to combi feed from when my baby was two days old and I was still in hospital. I'd had a difficult birth and was finding breastfeeding hard so decided to supplement with formula.' Samira

Intentionally using formula from birth

If you are planning to introduce some formula very early on, there are a few things to consider. Early breastfeeds are key to establishing a milk supply, which is necessary for breastfeeding to continue alongside formula. Furthermore, colostrum is a powerful and important substance, and it is definitely worth ensuring that your baby gets some of this if possible. Finally, the benefits of skin-to-skin time with your newborn baby are well-established as an important way to ease your baby's transition into the world, and time spent doing this is never wasted.[1]

Formula given at this stage should be in very small quantities, as larger amounts are likely to induce longer sleeps than are ideal, and will reduce the frequency with which the baby breastfeeds (and therefore take longer to establish the supply of breastmilk). As discussed in Chapter 3, this should be a first infant formula, safely prepared, and offered very slowly while paying attention to the baby so that they are not overwhelmed. You can get small pre-prepared bottles of formula milk for newborns, although these usually contain 70ml of milk, for a stomach that is accustomed to feeds of around 5–7ml, which may mean quite a lot of waste.

A newborn baby will breastfeed at least every 2–3 hours, so any time the breastfeed is replaced with formula, it will be helpful, if the mother can manage it, to try to express a small amount. This could then be used in place of the formula for some feeds. It could also be used to replace a breastfeed, but this again reduces the overall amount of breastfeeding, which will have an impact on the supply. Once the milk has come in, the mother may also need to express in order to prevent a build-up of milk or mastitis, and this will be discussed below under 'safely decreasing the supply'.

'I increased the amount of formula early, which was not the original plan.' Grace

Trying to manage two types of feeding together, while adjusting to life with your new baby, can be quite a lot of work. If you already have doubts about the likely success of breastfeeding, it can be very easy for the balance to tip towards using more formula, before you had planned for that to happen. For this reason, it may help to focus first on the breastfeeding, and give yourself at least a few days before bringing in the bottle, if you don't immediately need it.

As your baby grows, their appetite will increase. To maintain the breastmilk supply as they start to need more of it, they may sometimes ask to feed more frequently or for longer. The more you offer the breast, the longer you are likely to have breastmilk available as part of your feeding strategy. To maintain a balance, if the baby is taking more formula, then the breastmilk supply is likely to decrease.

Introducing formula milk after a few weeks

It is often suggested that parents might want to wait for a certain number of weeks before introducing a bottle. Rather than trying to specify a particular number of weeks, let's say that, if your focus in the first weeks is on establishing breastfeeding, then you can allow yourself the time and space to figure out how the bottle-feeds are going to fit in. You will be the best person to judge when the time is right, either to try expressing some milk, or to introduce some formula.

Think about how your day looks at the moment. Is there any sign of a predictable pattern yet? You may well still be feeding a lot, but do you have an idea about when your baby is likely to sleep, and for how long? This information will help you to identify times when you could express some milk, if that's your preference, and/or to allocate a time when the baby might have a bottle instead of a breastfeed. It is unlikely that your baby has very set feeding times, so it may be easier to choose a window of time (e.g. between 1pm and 4pm) when the baby could have the bottle. If someone else is going to be giving the bottle, talk to them about how this will work for both of you.

If you are going into this with breastfeeding well-established, then it will probably be necessary to express some milk around the time that the baby is having the bottle, to prevent a build-up of unneeded milk. If your plan is for the baby to have a bottle of *formula milk* at this time every day, then you only need to express a little bit to alleviate any engorgement, rather than enough milk to maintain the whole milk supply. This will then reduce the amount of milk available at that time (and can be reversed by breastfeeding or expressing more milk over a few days, if you change your mind).

If your plan is for the baby to have a bottle of *expressed milk* at this time every day, then you will need to continue expressing either at that time, or at other times during the day. In Chapter 4 we discussed different strategies for expressing, including pumping a small amount of milk at intervals during the day, and adding it together to make up one feed.

What if my baby refuses the bottle?

It is an anguish-inducing dilemma for parents, that they are told not to introduce a bottle too early in case their baby 'forgets' how to feed at the breast, but that if they don't introduce the bottle early enough, then the baby will 'refuse' to use it.

> *'I should have continued with a regular bottle when we stopped combi feeding as he then refused a bottle thereafter!'* Cat

We dealt with the idea of nipple confusion in Chapter 5, concluding that there is no evidence that using a bottle will undermine a baby's feeding reflexes. So now I am imagining your surprise when I reveal that there isn't any evidence for bottle refusal in older babies, either. Your three or four or five-month-old baby still doesn't have object permanence, and still can't plan to refuse the bottle and hold out for the breast. What they might do, instead, is find themselves being offered their milk in a strange new vessel that they simply don't know how to work, often in circumstances in which they are not entirely comfortable, such as being left with someone they don't know, or in an unfamiliar environment. A baby who is feeling out of sorts is in no position to learn a new skill, and given that they will often breastfeed for comfort, the bottle may seem like a preposterous alternative, and they might very much prefer a cuddle or a trip outside in a cosy sling.

It follows, then, that the best time to help your baby to learn how to use the bottle is when they are neither hungry nor distressed. Remember the paced bottle-feeding technique outlined in Chapter 5, which is thought to help babies to switch more easily between breast and bottle. And here are a few other hints and tips that might help:

- Sometimes a baby is more keen to take the bottle if it is offered in circumstances that are very similar to breastfeeding: from their mother or the parent who usually feeds them, held close to the body in a position that they normally feed in. If the mother is not available, you could try wrapping the bottle in something that smells like her (e.g. a muslin cloth).
- Sometimes the opposite is true, and it works better to make the breastfeed and the bottle-feed distinctly different: offered by someone else (with whom they feel comfortable), somewhere else, and in a very different position, or even moving around. Some mothers find that they actually need to leave the house before the bottle-feeding duo can properly get going.
- Offer the bottle when the baby is relaxed, not particularly hungry, and has their comfort needs met. And importantly, without the pressure of a deadline.
- Try warming the teat, or experimenting with different rates of flow.
- If the bottle contains expressed breastmilk, smell or taste it to check it doesn't taste funny. Occasionally the digestive enzyme lipase, which is present in breastmilk, causes the fats to start breaking down, and this can give rise to a soapy taste. The milk is safe for the baby, but they may not like it. If you are experiencing this, you can try scalding the milk immediately before storing it, which will stop the enzyme from working, and there are many websites that explain how to do this.[2]
- If your baby is getting closer to six months, there are some more alternatives to consider. You may find

that they manage better with a sippy cup or beaker, although you may have to hold it. Or they may be starting to have a little bit of solid food. And it's not unheard of for a baby to manage for several hours without a milk feed, and make up for it when reunited with their mother.

There is no official guidance on the best time to introduce a bottle to prevent bottle refusal. Nor is there any guarantee that a baby who takes a bottle early on will continue to do so later. This could be a tricky time for parents, but calm and patience usually help.

Short-term supplementation with formula or expressed breastmilk

Sometimes parents decide, or are encouraged, to offer supplements of formula or expressed breastmilk, or to 'top up' after a breastfeed. This usually happens if the baby is not feeding well at the breast, and there is an urgent need for them to have some milk. Parents may worry that the baby isn't getting enough milk at the breast, particularly if the baby seems unsettled or if they have very short or very long feeds; if this is your concern, do reach out for some specialist breastfeeding support or call one of the helplines to talk it through, as sometimes the challenge of coping with normal baby behaviour can undermine your confidence that breastfeeding is working.

If it is definitely the case that the baby is not getting enough milk at the breast, there will be some clear signs: fewer than two dirty nappies/5–6 wet nappies in 24 hours is the most obvious indication that a baby isn't feeding well. If they are feeding less than 10 times in 24 hours, and if they regularly sleep for very long periods (more than 4–5 hours at a time), this also might ring some alarm bells. It is important to look at the big picture of all these things together, as well as talking it through with a healthcare professional and/or a breastfeeding specialist.

> *'My baby lost a lot of weight and wasn't regaining it. After she got back to her birthweight, I stopped formula but she fussed at the breast a lot, causing me a lot of distress so we reintroduced top-ups and eventually, when she was six months old, she became purely formula fed as I had no milk left.'* Anna

At this point, you have a number of options, and may choose more than one of them:

- Seek specialist breastfeeding support to try to ascertain why the baby isn't feeding well, and then to help you resolve this
- Use any syringes of colostrum you have already collected
- Express some milk by hand or with a breast pump, and give this to the baby
- Request donor milk, if this is available
- Give the baby some formula milk

If, at this stage, your intention is to continue breastfeeding, then you will need specialist support alongside whatever other actions you decide to take. Remember what we said in Chapter 2 about the breastmilk supply: if the baby is having formula, then the mother will probably need to express to maintain her own milk supply until the issue with breastfeeding is resolved, when direct breastfeeding can resume. If she is able to express enough milk for the baby to have this instead of formula, this will generally be easier than trying to breastfeed AND express milk AND use formula – a situation known as 'triple feeding' that does not allow a great deal of time for rest and recovery from birth.

> *'Using formula as well as breastfeeding was a huge faff and inconvenience.'* Cat

How much and how often

It is impossible to generalise about how much milk a baby will need, if they are having an unknown amount at the breast, as well as a top-up of expressed milk or formula. The NHS talks about a total amount of milk equating to 150–200ml per kg of the baby's weight, for a baby under six months old.[3] You would need to divide this by roughly 12 feeds, and subtract the unknown amount that they are having at the breast... You see why it's tricky? This decision needs to take account of everything you and your health professionals know about how breastfeeding is going, to decide on the amount to give and the frequency with which to give it.

A healthy, full-term breastfeeding baby will usually feed 10–14 times in 24 hours, waking up to ask for feeds by signalling with their face and body. A baby who needs supplements will often be too sleepy to signal, so it may be appropriate to plan to feed the baby at maximum intervals, offering the feed as soon as they wake up, if this is earlier than the schedule dictates. A 2–3 hourly interval between feeds is normal, but – and I cannot emphasise this enough – *be led by your baby if they ask for a feed sooner than that.* There is nothing to be gained by delaying.

If you have some expressed milk available, offer this after a breastfeed, using the paced bottle-feeding method described in Chapter 5, allowing the baby plenty of breaks for their stomach to register fullness. If the plan also includes some formula, offer a small amount, again monitoring your baby to ensure you give plenty of breaks, and that they can control how much they take. Offering small amounts at frequent intervals is more closely aligned with what their body is able to manage, than large amounts at long intervals.

Increasing the amount of breastmilk

The amount of breastmilk available for the baby can be increased either by more direct breastfeeding, or more expressing. There are no foods that will increase your milk supply, as this is governed by your body's response to the amount of milk removed. Milk removal creates milk production, as we discussed in Chapter 2, so to increase the amount of milk being made, there are three key things you can do:

1. Increase the number of breastfeeds (or expressing sessions)
2. Ensure that you are feeding or expressing at least once in the night (levels of prolactin are highest between 2am and 6am)
3. Ensure your baby is feeding effectively: on cue, for as long as they wish to, and with a comfortable latch

'I felt fine initially as obviously she desperately needed it and at that point all we were interested in was getting her weight up and sodium down. But also a bit apprehensive of how we might revert back to just breastfeeding. Felt I had lost confidence a bit in my body to provide what she needed and started to rely on the formula safety net.'
Violet

Don't try to do all of this alone. There is so much support available for breastfeeding families, and most of it is free and should be geared up to helping you to achieve your stated goals.

> *'My daughter struggled to latch due to undiagnosed lip and tongue ties. I felt dreadful. I felt like a complete failure. I hated it. I wish I had known that there was help out there to get my daughter on the breast. Instead I pumped for her for five months alongside giving her formula.'* Ash

Decreasing the amount of breastmilk

If you have decided to move towards more formula, or to stop breastfeeding, you will need to consider how to do this in a way that does not cause you to become uncomfortably full, or to risk mastitis.

Depending on how many breastfeeds your baby is having over the course of a day, you may be able to stop quite quickly, or you may need to take a gradual approach. So if, for example, your baby only has one breastfeed in 24 hours, then you could stop that feed and keep an eye on how you feel physically; if you start to feel engorged, express just enough to feel comfortable, but no more.

If your baby is still having frequent breastfeeds, you *could* stop completely, but will need to be very vigilant about expressing as soon as you feel engorged, but again, just pumping enough to feel comfortable. Your body actually needs a small build-up of milk, so that this signals to the brain to stop making more of it. If you can avoid stopping so suddenly, a gradual weaning will be easier for your body, and quite probably easier for your baby to handle as well. Choose the feed that feels least important to you both (for example, a bedtime feed might still be very useful to you for settling your baby to sleep, so keep that one; or maybe that's precisely the one you are most looking forward to dropping – you get to choose!) When you are ready, stop offering that feed, replacing it with a bottle of expressed milk if you have that available, or formula. Notice if your breasts begin to feel full, and express a small amount. You will probably be able to express a bit less each time, until this no longer feels necessary.

It may be that the situation is not this straightforward. Perhaps your baby is having some solid food, or has started to sleep for longer without needing as many feeds. If you are happy that this means less breastfeeding, again, express as needed, and continue to monitor your baby's wellbeing by being aware of their levels of alertness, wet and dirty nappies, and growth and development.

Mastitis: what it is and what to do

Mastitis occurs when milk remains in the breast for longer than usual, which can happen for all sorts of reasons including the baby not having a good latch, and therefore not removing as much of it as they need. In this instance, we're talking about a situation where the milk remains in the breast because feeds are being replaced by formula milk.

The early signs of mastitis are usually a sore or lumpy patch in the breast, which may look darker than usual on light skin, and may feel hot to touch. Flu-like symptoms such as a temperature, aches and tiredness may then develop. Often if you attend to the early signs, you can avoid the flu symptoms. If you do get flu-like symptoms, then you may wish to see a GP for antibiotics.

When milk remains in the breast for longer than usual, an immune response causes inflammation, which then constricts the milk ducts, perpetuating the problem because it is then more difficult to remove the milk. Therefore your two-pronged approach to mastitis is to remove the milk and reduce the inflammation. The milk itself is not affected, and can be given to the baby. Because this is a situation where you do *not* intend to maintain the milk supply, you do not need to remove lots of milk, just enough to reduce the inflammation. You can do this as required.

Some other things that might help:

- Cool compresses (e.g. a damp flannel that has been in the fridge) to reduce inflammation
- Warm compresses to relieve pain and increase blood circulation
- Ibuprofen, if you can safely use this, or paracetamol
- Very gentle massage of the breast, towards the nipple. Doing this in the bath or shower can be particularly helpful
- Rest and fluids

Increasing supply again after it has decreased

What if you change your mind? Your body is highly adaptable. We know that if you breastfeed less, your milk supply will dip. Sometimes this happens after illness or a period of separation from your baby. The good news is that this can usually be reversed, by increasing the number of feeds or adding in some additional pumping. Very often, your baby will be more than willing to assist with this. Go back to Chapter 2 and refresh your understanding of how breastfeeding works, and – at the risk of sounding like a broken record – reach out for some skilled breastfeeding support. You don't have to do this on your own.

Babymoon

A strategy that can work very well is what's known as a 'babymoon.' Set aside a day, or even two, and ensure you have someone to look after you. Go to bed with your baby, or tuck yourself up on the sofa,* and cancel all other plans including visits from anyone you wouldn't breastfeed in front of. The role of the person looking after you is to bring you food and drinks, keep you company, and provide general reassurance that you really don't need to get up and do some tidying. Your role is to cuddle your baby, skin-to-skin as much as possible, and allow them unrestricted access to the breast. You may still need to offer additional expressed milk or formula, but prioritise breastfeeding. The skin contact alone can stimulate milk-producing hormones, and if the baby feeds very, very frequently, this too will encourage more milk to be produced. If this suggestion sounds like too much, you could pick a time of day when you feel able to do it for a few hours – a long morning lie-in, perhaps, or watching a movie in the evening.

Galactagogues

This marvellous word means a food or medication that increases the breastmilk supply. There are not very many, and using them would be a last resort, or at least something to do alongside skilled breastfeeding support that can explore all the other possible things you could try. In many cases, there is little or no evidence that food or medication is actually effective at increasing milk.

There is no evidence at all that oats or chocolate will increase your supply, and you do not have to drink milk to

---

* If you are spending time on the sofa, be very careful not to fall asleep with your baby, as this creates a higher risk of SIDS. If you are likely to fall asleep, you and your baby are safer in bed, providing the bed offers a firm, flat surface, and no bedding can tangle or smother the baby. Above all, do not sleep with your baby if you have been smoking or drinking alcohol.

make milk. You may find you are thirsty, so drink what you need to satisfy that thirst, but don't overdo it as over-hydration can be counter-productive. Any commercial or homemade 'lactation cookies' or breastfeeding teas are great if you like them, but they won't make the smallest difference to your ability to produce breastmilk.

There is limited evidence that herbs such as goat's rue, moringa and blessed thistle (also known as milk thistle) work, and only anecdotal reports that fenugreek may help. Herbal medicines may seem benign, but they are certainly not automatically safer than conventional medicine, and less is known about their side-effects.

The prescription medicines domperidone and metoclopramide, which are used to treat nausea and vomiting, have been shown to increase prolactin levels, and therefore to increase breastmilk production. In *Why Mothers' Medication Matters*, Dr Wendy Jones[4] describes these as safe, with insignificant transfer into the milk; however, they are not licensed for this use, and therefore it can be difficult to get GPs to prescribe them. The Breastfeeding Network website has a good factsheet that might be worth sharing with your health professional if you are considering this approach. Wendy goes on to point out that effective breastfeeding, and good breastfeeding support, are still likely to be more helpful.[5]

Mixed feeding in hot weather

Caring for a newborn in a heatwave can bring up all sorts of additional challenges, including that your baby, like you, will be hot, thirsty and uncomfortable. All of the usual hot weather advice applies to both of you: dress lightly, stay in the shade, stay hydrated and so on. Your baby may well be unsettled and asking for a *lot* of extra feeds. You have some options to consider:

1. Offer more breastfeeds

When babies breastfeed very frequently, breastmilk tends to have a higher water content, which will hydrate them as required. If they feed more frequently than usual, your body may respond by increasing the amount of milk made. This could be helpful if you are trying to increase your supply, or unhelpful if not (see the above sections on increasing/decreasing the amount of breastmilk, for how to manage this).

2. Offer small amounts of cooled, boiled water

This would be in addition to their regular feeds. Do not replace any milk feeds with water, as this will result in your baby missing out on important nutrients. If your baby seems to be taking very large amounts of water, then it may be that they do in fact need more milk to support their growth and development. This can feel like a tricky balancing act, so do please talk to your health visitor or seek support from a breastfeeding counsellor, to help you decide on the right thing to do.

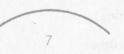

7

Mixed Feeding
Twins and Multiples

by Janet Rimmer

Janet is an NCT Breastfeeding Counsellor and a mother of 26-year-old triplets whom she breastfed. For the last 10 years she has trained and supported a team of NCT breastfeeding peer supporters for Twins Trust, who offer mother-to-mother feeding support and information to other parents of multiples.

The first thing to say, up front, is that breastfeeding is an option as available to parents of multiples as it is to parents of singletons. This might seem a strange place to start a chapter on mixed feeding and formula use with twin and triplet children, but here's why I've done it.

Two key cultural messages can influence the decisions parents of twin and triplet babies take about mixed feeding and formula use and these need to be exposed and examined.

Firstly, there is a general myth which floats around that says that mothers of twins and triplets are unlikely to be able to produce enough breastmilk to feed two or three babies and therefore are less able to achieve their feeding goals than parents of singletons. Following on from this is the idea that parents of multiples should aim to mix feed their babies, which is commonly suggested from the moment a twin and especially a triplet pregnancy is confirmed. This myth can be reinforced by those who have never seen breastfeeding twins and do not have confidence in what women can achieve. Starting the feeding journey with the thought that fully breastfeeding twins or triplets is unlikely or impossible can mean that if things become challenging it can reinforce that idea, so may lead to the introduction of formula milk not through choice, but from a feeling of inevitability.

However, many mothers of twins and triplets do achieve their goals, be it to breastfeed for a day, a week, a month or a year and longer. The research that has been done into women feeding twins and triplets suggests that mothers often report worries about their milk supply, but this can be seen as a response to the doubts raised in their minds rather than an inability to produce enough milk. A systematic review of the available evidence found that 'most women can produce sufficient breastmilk to breastfeed multiples' (Multiple Births Foundation, 2011). Breastmilk production is based on the supply and demand mechanism, and therefore it is possible to cater for the needs of more than one baby (see Chapter 2), provided the support is there to breastfeed babies in response to their needs.

There are things which can disrupt a mother's breastmilk supply, and twins and triplet babies and parents are more prone to some than singletons (such as the challenges connected with premature birth), but the logical response to this fact is to increase the level of support offered to parents of multiples rather than tell them it's best not to try.

The second thing to say is that you do not need to be a superwoman to achieve your goal if that is to breastfeed your twins or triplets. This is another myth which is perpetuated and can undermine a woman's belief in her own ability to breastfeed. It does help if it is something you are motivated to do, and it also really helps if you have informed support around you to achieve that goal, but superwoman? Nah. That's optional. For the last 10 years I have worked with a group of women who trained as peer supporters because of their experience of hearing that message and still breastfeeding their babies. These women are remarkable in their desire to support others and their willingness to give up their precious time to do it. However, each of them has a story to tell about their feeding journey and all have had challenges on the way.

As discussed elsewhere in this book, using some formula milk can either support your breastfeeding or chestfeeding journey or undermine it. It can be a way of continuing your breastfeeding journey when you are feeling overwhelmed and wondering if you will ever sleep again for more than 30 minutes at a go, or it can undermine any confidence you can feel in your body's ability to produce milk which will satisfy and grow your babies. I am going to draw on the experiences of the many parents I have spoken to over the years who have used a mixture of breastmilk and formula milk to feed their babies and pick out some of the themes, ideas and actions that have emerged about what made it work for them. And that is the key point in all of this. It's what works for you as a parent.

Making mixed feeding work for your family

The experience of many parents of twins and triplets is that they look for information on feeding multiple babies and find information on feeding single babies and adapt it. If there is anything added in, it's about routines and positions for feeding two babies at once. Sometimes that's okay, but at other times it can feel as if the author doesn't understand what it means to have two or three babies all needing to be responded to individually, or that each parent of multiples will want to feed their babies in the way that suits them. Taking advice based on caring for one baby and adapting it to two or more can lead to complicated and unsustainable routines. Feeding two or more babies can require imagination and creativity. Most of all it means understanding who you want to be as a parent rather than just counting the number of babies and following a plan.

Feeding each baby in a different way

It is not unusual for twin or triplet babies to be very different in their ability to feed from the breast and in their needs for milk. As will happen throughout their lives, twin and triplet children hit different milestones at different times and in different ways. One of the opportunities offered by having twin babies is to mix and match when it comes to feeding. If one baby is struggling to feed effectively at the breast, feeding alongside their more effective twin can help the milk flow. Swapping breasts so the more effective feeder can stimulate both breasts can be a useful option for getting the breastmilk supply established in the early days. If one baby is struggling to attach, the other can keep the milk supply going until they are more able to do so. In that situation feeding one baby and expressing from the other breast can enable the second baby to have expressed breastmilk.

It can happen that one baby continues to struggle at the breast, and it makes sense to the parents that they continue to feed that baby using a bottle. This can be expressed milk or formula milk or a mixture of both. Sometimes parents wonder about whether it is fair to the baby who is receiving formula milk for their sibling/siblings to receive breastmilk. They can worry that they may bond less with the child who is bottle-fed. If expressing becomes too challenging to fit into their day and the baby receives formula milk in their bottle, then some parents can make the decision to stop all breastfeeding. This is one of the constant challenges as a parent of multiples: responding to each child's individual needs while being fair to them all.

Fair doesn't mean equal

It can be useful to think about the idea of twin or triplet children as needing different things at different times in their lives. Fair doesn't necessarily mean equal and so there will be times when your children will receive different things from you at different times. For example, as they get older, if one child is interested in football and another is not keen on sport, then you may decide to spend time with the other child while your first child heads to the pitch. You may wish they were both potential Lionesses, but you won't stop one because the other misses the ball every time they swing for it. As has been discussed elsewhere (Chapter 5), close and loving feeding can be done when feeding from a bottle and can enable you to build a loving relationship with your baby. If as a breastfeeding mother you feel distressed about what your second child is missing, then bringing that baby to the breast when the other baby feeds can enable the first baby to have a few drops expressed into their mouth and the same close contact. Even if babies don't take the majority of their milk from their mother's breast they can still stay there and be comforted and attach themselves if they and their mother wish.

Here are some ideas of ways you can take this forward:

	Pros	Cons
One parent breastfeeds one or two, the other baby is fed by the other parent or regular supporter with bottle	Clearly defined roles and an established pattern	Parents may feel less connected to opposite baby
The breastfeeding parent feeds whichever baby is indicating they need to feed first with their allocated method then feeds the second baby afterwards then the third baby if there is one	Parent who is feeding the babies has time to respond individually to each baby	A feeding cycle can take a long time especially when the babies are smaller
The breastfeeding parent also feeds the baby with a bottle at the same time with the baby cuddled up or on a cushion next to her or with both on a feeding cushion	This becomes easier as the mother becomes more confident	Can be challenging to focus on attaching the first baby while feeding the second.
Baby breastfeeds while the other baby is finger fed or fed at the breast with a supplemental nursing system (SNS)	Mother can feed both babies at the same time	Some parents find supplemental feeding fiddly to get established
Both parents lactate and both bottle and breastfeed as needed	Can be a very flexible way to share feeding for mothers and babies	The non-pregnant parent will need support and information to induce lactation

Sharing the bottle-feeds around

Some parents decide that they want to introduce some bottle-feeds and share them among the babies so that all the babies have some breastmilk and some formula milk. In this scenario it can be helpful to establish breastfeeding first with all babies and then gradually introduce the bottles. Which brings me on to the next question...

When should we start introducing a bottle of formula?

Elsewhere in this book (Chapter 6) the idea of establishing the breastmilk supply first then adding in formula milk has been discussed. If this is possible it remains a good option for a family planning to mix feed over several months.

However, for many twin parents, introducing a bottle of formula isn't a choice but rather something which happens in response to circumstances. This is typically the case if babies are born early and need encouragement to feed while being given additional food in the form of expressed breastmilk or formula milk. Moving towards breastfeeding takes time and so, when there are overstretched resources in a hospital unit, there can be encouragement from staff for parents to feed their babies with bottles in order to be discharged home. The challenge can be that parents wishing to fully breastfeed their babies are discharged home with a regime of offering the breast, then giving breast or formula milk top-ups after each feed and then expressing for the next feed. This scenario can mean that for the lactating parent with two or three babies, the entire feeding episode can lead to little time to have a break or a rest before the next feeding cycle starts. For many mothers it becomes unsustainable and the road to fully feeding with formula beckons.

A note to health professionals

If your team is discharging mothers home with their babies on a feeding regime it would really help parents to have, as part of the plan, a review whereby mothers are supported to move to a more sustainable way of feeding their babies once they are putting on sufficient weight. I have met mothers who have continued with hospital regimes when their babies are piling on weight and have been given no information about how they can make the transition to either fully breastfeeding or to a more efficient way of mixed feeding their babies.

Babies born at full-term

Multiple-birth babies who are born at 37 weeks or later are considered full-term. They typically have a lower birth weight than single babies and it is very common to hear they are sleepy and need quite a bit of encouragement to feed in the early weeks. It is possible that, in this scenario, concerns about the babies taking sufficient milk will lead to the suggestion that the parents add top-ups of formula milk to every feed. How this is enacted requires some thought so that breastfeeding can continue. Techniques like breast compressions can enable babies to take more breastmilk from the breast at each feed.[2] Paced bottle-feeding, if adding in top-ups, can also be helpful. Empowering parents to have the confidence to drop top-ups as their babies take more milk is a key part of the picture.

Paced bottle-feeding with twins and triplets

If babies are to be fed with a bottle the guidance given now from respected sources is to pace the feeds and feed responsively.[3] The guidance encourages parents to follow their baby's cues to feed and slow the feeds down using a slow teat and pauses in the feeding. Cuddling up with one baby can be an option if there are others around to share each feed, but many parents, if not all, will have times when they will be feeding on their own.

If you have people feeding your babies from the bottle you may need to introduce them to this method and ask them to keep to the approach. Older generations may not be familiar with this idea, and so it may be challenging to assert your ideas when you are dependent on their support. Sharing information such as the *NHS Guide to Bottle-feeding*[4] can explain what you are trying to achieve.

If you need to feed two together using bottles, then deciding on one or two areas in your home where you can feed both babies can be a useful idea. You can set things up there, experimenting with cushions and ways to sit so you can see and respond to both babies.

Firstly, think about yourself. You are going to be sitting with your babies for a while so you will need to be comfortable. Where could you sit that gives you space on both sides on the same level as you? Create a nest around yourself to feel well supported and to support your arms. Then place the babies within arms' reach, enabling you to have eye contact with each of them. The closer they are to you, and the closer together they are, the easier it is to keep observing their cues. Your babies may be in bouncy chairs or bean bags or propped up by carefully chosen cushions. Some specialist twin-feeding cushions allow babies to be supported more upright on one side and to lie flat on the other, or you could prop a pillow/cushion underneath the far side of the feeding cushion so the pillow tips up and the babies sit more upright inside the cushion close to you. Think about what happens when one stops feeding: will you be able to have one over your shoulder while the other continues feeding? Can you have a bouncy chair there to keep them upright? Or cushions to support them? They may need less winding than you think. Creating a nest will enable the babies to be upright once they have finished feeding and you may wish to keep your hand on their body so the contact between you remains. Check you have all you need nearby in case one possets or you need a drink.

Finding a pattern to your day

Though I have spoken with parents who are happy to let their babies dictate the pace and prefer the experience of responding to each baby individually, many parents of multiples are searching for a pattern to their day which has some predictability. I have also met parents who feel they should have a pattern because that's what everyone has told them they need, but it's causing them more stress trying to maintain it. So you may wish to consider who you are as a parent and how, and whether, you want to create a pattern in your days. Once you understand that, you can follow what works for you.

In the first few days and weeks it is not uncommon for premature babies newly discharged from hospital to be sleepy and to seem to have fallen into a pattern quite happily, often one suggested by the hospital staff. This can often be the case for twin babies born at 37+ weeks. As the babies grow, they can become more alert and patterns of feeding change. This can be a time to rethink and re-evaluate what might work for you and your family. You might try keeping a note of when they feed and whether they are feeding together. Then start to think about when the best time might be to introduce a bottle of formula milk. Knowing a support person will be available at that time may be a deciding factor, as might your tiredness levels and willingness to try something new. When might it suit you and your babies?

	Pros	Cons
Feeding one (or two) babies and rotating the other one with a feed from the bottle	Each baby gets some breastmilk and the lactating parent gets to spend time with each of them at the breast	With small babies the times between babies wanting to feed can vary and synchronising the feeds can be tricky
Breastfeeding all babies for most feeds then choosing one or two times when they all have a paced bottle-feed	If the times are chosen when support is available, then the mother can have a break from feeding and look to self-care	Can be tiring to feed two or three babies from the bottle if support is not available, so it may not give the mother the break she was hoping for
Offering the breast to each baby and then adding in a top-up of formula milk for each baby who shows signs of needing more milk	This may be a valid short-term approach when babies are unable to feed actively long enough to take on sufficient food	This approach tends to be unsustainable other than as a short-term measure, though some families can and do continue when sufficient support is available

Getting the support you need

It can be hard to find support for feeding multiple babies. One mother of triplets recounted that when seeking support for feeding her babies she felt frustrated that instead of a conversation focused on offering her ideas, she received a barrage of questions, and comments on how amazing it was that she was feeding all three. She told me that she came away without any of the practical support she needed. Some parents do appreciate encouragement and recognition of their achievements, but as well as and not instead of practical support.

There are sources of support especially for parents of multiples and places you can meet other mothers of twin and triplet children. There is an active Facebook community which has been set up by the charity Breastfeeding Twins and Triplets UK. The group and website provide some excellent information and support for parents of multiples on feeding two or three babies.

Twins Trust has a group of mothers trained by the NCT as peer supporters who have breastfed their babies and are happy to talk with you about your challenges. More importantly they are trained to listen carefully to your concerns, without judgement, and then share the information you decide you need (or point you in the direction of where to find it). They will do this on a one-to-one basis, or you can join the weekly drop-in with other parents of multiples to discuss all things feeding related.

Notes to supporters

I am often asked what should be shared with parents of multiples about feeding twins and triplets by those who are searching for the right information to unlock the door to successful feeding. I find that behind that question is the idea that having breastfed triplets, I have knowledge of what will work for all parents of twins and triplets. I can tell you categorically that this isn't the case. And that's because we are not all the same. We have some things in common, yes, and there's a common understanding between us of the challenges we face with two or more babies, but families of multiples are as diverse as families of singletons and will need a full range of support. Many will be older parents as the chances of conceiving two or more increase with age,[5] while many gay and lesbian couples become parents of multiples through fertility treatments which have an increased rate of multiple pregnancies.[6] Some communities have higher rates of twins than others.[7] There are families who considered and hoped for the possibility of twins, and there are families for whom twins (and triplets) come out of the blue and they are left reeling from shock and counting the seats in their family car. Each family will experience a range of emotions on finding out they are expecting twins or triplets: some total and utter joy, some complete horror and every other emotion in between. All will be considered high-risk pregnancies,[8] and parents may start their feeding journeys concerned about their babies' milk intake from day one. Some may have waited years and have doubted they will ever become parents. Some will have other singleton children and may bring a wealth of experience as parents.

For all those who support parents of multiples and their feeding journeys I offer this suggestion: look past the number of babies and see the mother or lactating parent. Listen to them and what they want and how they feel. Share ideas and, if you are not sure, be prepared to say so and offer to be alongside them while you work it out together. They will each know what will work for them and what won't, and they will appreciate the space to consider ideas with you.

A note on the reality of parenting multiples

The reality of parenting two or three babies can be very different from what is imagined. Few parents anticipate a multiple pregnancy. Though the number of multiple pregnancies following IVF has reduced significantly since

2007, for some there may have been a significant period of time between the thought of wanting a child to holding their babies in their arms. Over half of twins and all triplets and more babies are born early, many requiring some time in neonatal care, and twins born at 37+ weeks are still smaller and usually sleepier than their singleton peers. Consequently, when the babies are born there can be a significant gap in parents' minds between the idea of their babies and the reality of caring for two or more. Perhaps unsurprisingly, parents of multiples are thought to be more vulnerable to postnatal depression.[9] Those who have had a long journey to conception and birthing their children can feel unable to talk about how hard parenting is in case they are perceived as ungrateful.[10] Their journey to parenthood cannot be divorced from the feeding experience. Anxiety about their babies' weight can fuel their decisions without informed support. Lest this sounds unduly gloomy, there is a great deal of joy as well. The pride parents can feel in their parenting is immense. The pleasure of seeing their children interact and grow is enormous. The unique anxieties and joys of parenting three babies are eloquently and entertainingly explored in the three-part podcast by Cole Moreton 'The Power of Three'.

Links for twin feeding support

Twins Trust provides support for all parents of multiples at all stages of their parenting journey. This includes an NCT-trained group of women who offer mother-to-mother support to all mothers and parents whether fully breastfeeding, fully formula feeding or anything in between.

They offer the opportunity via email, phone or text for mothers to talk through their feeding challenges and explore their options without being judged. And in a weekly drop-in they have the opportunity to share experiences in a supportive environment with other mothers and parents of multiples.

Breastfeeding Twins and Triplets UK provides information in a series of twin and triplet-focused blog posts by Kathryn Stagg, IBCLC. In addition it hosts an active Facebook group to support UK-based breastfeeding parents nursing twins or triplets: **breastfeedingtwinsandtriplets.co.uk**

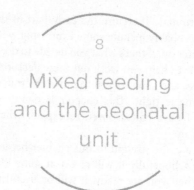

8

Mixed feeding and the neonatal unit

This chapter is specifically about the experience of mixed feeding a baby who is sick or premature, and needs to spend time in the neonatal unit (NNU).

If you are in this situation, you may not have started to think much about feeding your baby yet, or your plans and expectations may have had to change dramatically. It is likely that you are worried about your baby, and the birth itself may also have been difficult or even traumatic. You may have known that your baby would need this extra care, and be reading this chapter in preparation.

It is very likely that your baby will receive a combination of fluids and expressed colostrum to start with, moving on from fluids as they get stronger. It is very unlikely that they will be able to have formula milk under 32 weeks, because of the risk of a condition called necrotising enterocolitis (NEC), which is discussed below (although in hospitals with access to donor human milk, this may be given to babies under 34 weeks instead of formula). Therefore the early part of this feeding journey will probably include some expressing, with formula introduced later on, if that's what you decide to do. NNU staff should be able to help you work out these decisions, support you to express, and support you to move on from expressing when the time is right. This chapter is dauntingly full of initials, and I have endeavoured to explain what all these acronyms mean.

If you have come straight to this chapter because of your circumstances, hopefully it will give you some idea of what to expect. When you are ready, it will be useful to go back to some earlier sections of the book, especially Chapter 2 on breastfeeding and Chapter 4 on expressing. You might be about to encounter some or all of the things I describe below, not necessarily in this order, and there should be someone available to talk through each stage of the process with you.

Reasons your baby might be in the neonatal unit

According to BLISS (the charity for premature and sick babies), one in seven babies need neonatal care. The main reasons for NNU admission are premature birth (before 37 weeks of pregnancy), low birth weight (under 2.5kg/5lb), or where the baby has a medical condition that requires treatment.

Prematurity covers a range starting from 'extremely premature' babies born before 28 weeks of gestation, with some units looking after babies as young as 23 weeks. The ability to coordinate sucking and swallowing with breathing normally develops around 34–36 weeks (sometimes earlier), so an extremely premature baby is likely to need a lot of help to feed.

Initially, these babies may not be ready to digest milk, and will be fed with total parenteral nutrition (PN), often referred to just as 'fluids', given intravenously. PN contains vitamins, minerals, protein, carbohydrates, and fats. As the baby gets stronger, this will gradually be replaced by milk feeds, given by a tube through the nose or mouth.

Low birth weight is often part of the picture when a baby is premature. It can also happen when growth has slowed or stopped during pregnancy. Twins or multiple babies often have low birth weight (see Chapter 7). Babies with low birth weight are more likely to have health conditions including infections, difficulty breathing, and difficulty digesting milk, and therefore will need neonatal care until their condition improves.

Medical conditions can range from relatively mild and treatable conditions such as jaundice, to much more severe conditions where the baby needs life support. Babies may also be admitted to NNU for observation after a difficult birth, or if they are awaiting surgery for a known issue.

What to expect in the NNU

There are different levels of neonatal care, depending on your baby's needs. This will vary slightly from hospital to hospital, and sometimes it may be necessary for the baby to transfer to a different hospital, if their needs cannot be met at the hospital where they were born. The set-up will usually be something like this:

Neonatal Intensive Care Unit (NICU) is for the babies needing the most medical care – those who are very premature, or have serious breathing difficulties.

Some hospitals will have a *Neonatal High Dependency Unit (HDU)* for babies who do not need intensive care. Babies who have been in NICU will move on to the HDU as their condition improves.

From here, babies will move to the *Low Dependency Unit (LDU)* or *Special Care Baby Unit (SCBU)*, or they may be admitted here for monitoring or help with less complex or severe conditions. Often babies are discharged from SCBU, but some hospitals have a *Transitional Care Unit* where the baby might stay together with the parents and then go home.

The BLISS website has a wealth of information about what to expect from the NNU (bliss.org.uk); we are going to focus specifically on feeding.

The importance of breastmilk

Breastmilk and particularly colostrum are important in this situation. Colostrum has a protective effect against infection, and contains a high concentration of hormones and proteins that stimulate growth. If the baby is being tube-fed PN, they will also be given drops of colostrum orally (known as buccal colostrum). Research shows that colostrum given to very low birth weight babies within 12 hours of birth reduces the risk of sepsis and a condition called necrotising enterocolitis (NEC), and reduces the time taken for the babies to move from PN to full milk feeds.[1]

When babies are born prematurely, the composition of breastmilk is slightly different from full-term breastmilk, with higher concentrations of certain nutrients such as proteins and fats.[2] This will support your baby's energy requirements, but they may need an additional fortifier in certain circumstances, to help them to grow.

Necrotising enterocolitis (NEC)

This is a serious condition in which the tissues of the baby's intestines become inflamed. This can make babies extremely unwell, sometimes requiring surgery to remove part of the gut, and it can be fatal. Premature babies, whose digestive systems are not sufficiently mature to digest milk, are more at risk of this condition, which is one of the reasons they will be given PN rather than milk at first.

Breastmilk can offer some protection against NEC,[3] but if the condition develops, milk feeds will usually be stopped in order to rest the bowel, and the baby will go back to having PN. This means that the balancing act of moving from PN to milk feeds can be a delicate one. Medical staff on NNU are highly attuned to the signs of NEC and are likely to act quickly if symptoms appear.

The importance of breastmilk for your sick or premature baby means that you will be encouraged to express breastmilk as soon as possible, both to establish a supply of milk, and so that it can be given to the baby.

Donor milk is available in some hospitals, for sick or premature babies where their mother's own breastmilk is not available. Human milk banks usually serve their local region. Milk is collected, screened and pasteurised before being distributed to those babies who need it the most. This means that formula milk can be avoided, and babies can receive the protective and growth-supporting effects of breastmilk. For more information, you can look at the UK Association of Milk Banks (ukamb.org) and the Human Milk Foundation (humanmilkfoundation.org).

Expressing milk for your baby in NNU

Chapter 4 covers what you need to know about expressing, so here we will focus on the particular challenges of doing this in the NNU, and how it might feel.

Expressing breastmilk means that your baby can have some of this important substance alongside PN, and will also be the first step towards establishing a supply of milk, meaning that this option remains open to you. Therefore midwives are likely to support you to start expressing as early as possible, usually within the first two hours after the birth, and to express around 8–10 times in 24 hours, including once at night. Depending on their health and development, from around 34 weeks you will also be encouraged to put your baby to the breast for a bit of a nuzzle around, which will begin to help with stimulation of the milk supply, and perhaps trigger some feeding reflexes in the baby.

The NNU is a physically and emotionally stressful place, and whatever your birth was like, you will now be recovering from that experience. You may not be able to stay with your baby, in which case you will be on a postnatal ward, or even at home. If your baby has been transferred to a hospital further away from your home, you may be spending a lot of time travelling to be with them.

Inevitably, this creates challenges for expressing, which works best in a relaxed, oxytocin-rich environment. It is important to acknowledge that this is what is going on for you, and be prepared only to produce a tiny amount of colostrum the first few times you do this. These valuable drops will be given to your baby alongside the PN.

Initially, the midwives will support you to express colostrum by hand. If this is not happening, you can ask to see an infant feeding specialist, who will have specific training in supporting mothers to start breastfeeding. There is evidence that early pumping can increase the overall yield of milk,[4] so best practice is to begin hand-expressing colostrum in the first two hours, using heat and massage of the breast prior to doing this, and then to pump for five minutes on each side to stimulate production.

As your milk starts to change and increase in quantity, after a few days, you might then start to use a breast pump more often. This should be provided for you by the hospital, and the NNU usually has an expressing room that you can use. In her memoir of giving birth to premature twins *Mothership*, Francesca Segal[5] describes this room – 'the milking shed' – as a place where she learns and receives support from the other expressing mothers, who share their experience and compare their babies' progress. However, some mothers find that higher milk volumes are produced when expressing at the cot side, so you may wish to check if it is possible for you to do this.

The focus of your expressing in these first few days is to build up a supply of milk, and this is likely to happen slowly – and, while your baby is having PN, that's okay. You do not urgently have to produce large volumes of expressed milk, as your baby's stomach capacity is tiny, and even the smallest quantities will benefit them alongside the PN. Be aware that you will get differing amounts at different times; if you have had a difficult day, or there has been a change in your baby's routine, then there might be less milk expressed the following day. For this reason, it can be helpful to look at the volume produced over 24 hours, rather than to focus on what you manage to get at individual expressing sessions. Try not to panic, do as much as you feel you can manage, and when you feel a bit better, then do a bit more. Give yourself a break when you need it.

If it is possible to hold your baby, then having them skin-to-skin on your chest as much as you feel able to or allowed to, can have great benefits for both of you. Skin-to-skin contact with your body supports your baby's growth, regulates their temperature, heartrate, breathing, oxygen saturations, and blood sugars; contributes to the development and balancing of their microbiome and reduces their stress. In addition, skin-to-skin time is linked to increased yield of expressed milk. NNU staff will help you to have skin-to-skin with your baby/ies. Being able to touch and hold your baby can shorten their hospital stay, and make you feel less stressed.

'Skin-to-skin for neonatal babies is magic.' Louise Oliver, Neonatal Infant Feeding Advisor

Other things that can help to increase your yield are visualising yourself holding or feeding your baby, having a piece of their clothing or bedding with their smell, or a picture of them, or being close to them if this is possible. It might be worth experimenting with a different size of pump flange, if you're finding expressing uncomfortable or ineffective. Remember: do what you can. Anxiety about how much you can produce will be counter-productive, and your baby will be getting fluids while you gradually build your supply. Celebrate every drop.

Moving on

As your baby's condition improves, staff on the ward will discuss with you the appropriate next steps, and will monitor your baby's progress with you. These conversations will be highly tailored to your situation, so rather than trying to cover every eventuality, my suggestion is to ask questions, take notes, and have someone there to support you in working things out. Your options at this point will be largely based on what your baby can do, and how much breastmilk is available, but remember that none of this is fixed and permanent.

As with most aspects of feeding babies, this is a hugely individual experience. You may never have planned to breastfeed, and yet now have enough milk to feed the whole ward. Or perhaps you really wanted to breastfeed, but the circumstances have been stacked against you, and you haven't yet established a milk supply sufficient to meet all of your baby's or babies' calculated feeding requirements.

You may be ready to stop expressing, especially if you strongly associate expressing milk with the whole neonatal unit experience: closing the door of the expressing room, or handing back your loaned pump, could be an important part of moving on from the NNU. Acknowledging that you don't want to express anymore does not make you a bad mother.

> *'Don't make the decision to stop on a bad day.'* Gillian Denton, Neonatal Feeding Lead at Oxford University Hospitals NHS Trust

The same applies if you have been breastfeeding, and now decide not to continue. Your milk has seen your baby through the first difficult days or weeks of their life; celebrate what you've achieved in such challenging circumstances.

Formula and bottles

From about 34 weeks, you might introduce formula milk either because there is an insufficient supply of breastmilk, or because you decide that you want to. This does not have to be your final decision, and could be a temporary or transitional decision, for example where the baby needs to be feeding enough to go home. In Chapter 6 we explored ways of managing breastfeeding alongside formula, and, in addition to reading this, you may be able to access different forms of breastfeeding support outside the hospital.

If your plan is to continue with some breastfeeding alongside formula, it can be helpful to offer the breast or expressed breastmilk first, and to continue having skin-to-skin time with your baby, to stimulate milk production and ensure that any breastmilk available is used. In fact, all tube and bottle-feeds could be done at the breast, which again stimulates milk production.

If your baby is also tube-feeding, the recommendation is to offer the breast at some feeds and the bottle at others, but not to try to do all three at the same feed. Gillian Denton describes this as 'too much for the baby', but I can imagine it being a lot for parents to manage as well.

If this is the first time you have used bottles, staff should support you to learn about paced bottle-feeding (see Chapter 5), and prioritise you as the parents to give the bottle whenever you are around, as practice and as an opportunity to hold your baby as much as possible. Remember, skin-to-skin is magic. Be prepared to go very slowly with these early bottles, using a suitable teat designed for premature babies (i.e. a very slow flow teat). Allow your baby plenty of breaks, and if they cannot finish the feed by bottle (or breast), the nasogastric tube can be used to provide the rest.

Transitioning to the breast

A baby who has been tube-fed can usually start practising their breastfeeding skills at around 31–34 weeks, as those reflexes start to develop, and they are getting stronger. Initially, this can be a continuation of that magic skin-to-skin time, simply offering them the opportunity to nuzzle around. Hold your baby in a position that they enjoy, and which is comfortable for you – perhaps reclining with plenty of back support, and starting with them lying on your body with their head near the breast. This full body contact can trigger feeding reflexes, and your baby might like to search around, interested by what they can see, smell and feel. Keep them calm, and try to enjoy the moment even if they don't do very much at this stage.

Over the next few days, perhaps they will do a little bit more. Remember that you have other means of feeding them, and this time is best spent with both of you learning about how it all fits together.

Moving on from NNU

Once your baby is well enough to go home, the bar that you have to reach with feeding is either that they can bottle-feed (breastmilk and/or formula milk), or that you and they can manage at least two good breastfeeds per day alongside tube-feeding. This means they can go home still tube-feeding, but if for some reason the tube is pulled out, you will still be able to feed them until the tube is fixed. This requires an adequate milk supply, effective latch, consistent weight gain, and good nappy output. Your baby should be feeding at least eight times in 24 hours, as responsively as possible – that is, feed them when they signal that they would like to be fed, and feed them proactively in addition to this if necessary.

Life after NNU could feel like both an ending and a beginning, and you may still wish to access support now that you're out in the community. Your midwife and then your health visitor will be making themselves available to you, and you will have access to the same support discussed in Chapter 9, like anyone else who needs help with feeding a baby.

Thanks to Louise Oliver, Neonatal Infant Feeding Advisor and Breastfeeding Counsellor at Birmingham Women's Hospital NNU; and Gillian Denton, Neonatal Feeding Lead at Oxford University Hospitals NHS Trust.

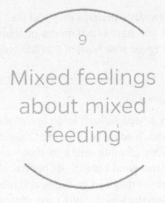

9

Mixed feelings about mixed feeding

At the beginning of this book, I wrote about the complex circumstances in which parents make decisions about feeding their babies, and set out my plan to try and make things a little bit easier. I hope that, on a practical level, there has been some useful information for you. I fear that, in an emotional sense, we may not have come very far. This chapter is about the range of feelings that parents have when they introduce formula, whether that's always been part of the plan, or an unexpected development.

For some people, it goes without a hitch, and even then, this feels like a stroke of luck. And it does indeed seem lucky, in today's society, to make a parenting decision, stick to it, and feel no doubt that it was the right one for your family. Yet I can't help thinking that that should be the minimum we hope for.

'I hoped to breastfeed with a baby [who] took the bottle as an alternative. I was very happy about this as it couldn't have gone better. I felt we were very lucky.' Marie

Even when this is a wholly positively planned and implemented decision, there can be some mixed feelings.

'I felt a bit guilty, like I was putting myself before my child. I think this stemmed from the enforced message from society and NHS that breastmilk is best and a stigma is created around formula feeding.' Grace

For any of this to change, we need to move on from the divisive narrative of breast v bottle, laden with moral judgement and devoid of compassion or understanding of women's lived experience of feeding their babies in 21st-century Britain, where breastfeeding rates are already the lowest in the world, and parents feel unprepared, unsupported, and judged *no matter how they feed their babies.*[1]

'I didn't feel prepared at all – had naively planned to just breastfeed so we didn't have any of the bottles etc and didn't know how much baby would need. I didn't feel very supported at the hospital because they just said the baby would get nipple confusion (this never happened and I ended up mixed feeding until my baby was 10 months).' Samira

Before the birth

We are exposed to the breastfeeding culture war long before we become parents, and come to motherhood full of doubts and anxieties. Author Naomi Stadlen[2] points out that 'uncertainty is a good starting point for a mother,' acknowledging that we each have to figure out how to do this for ourselves. Even with the best role models, our families and our parenting will be unique to us. What can you do with all this uncertainty? Two things, really: firstly, get informed, think about what you want, and try to understand how that works. Undoubtedly you will have to adapt this knowledge once you meet your baby, and have to navigate the reality of new parenthood. Secondly, find your team. Surround yourself with people who have got your back, who understand what you want, and will champion that. Breastfeeding counsellors and peer supporters, despite the title, can be among those people. You may also have family and friends who will be on your side; and this is a good reason to include your partner or someone who will be supporting you after the birth, in any antenatal course you go along to.

During pregnancy, you may become aware of pressures in both directions, as well as advice that inevitably involves mixed feeding (we discussed 'make sure they take a bottle' in Chapter 5). Remember that you don't have to make a decision at this stage, but that knowing a bit about breastfeeding will keep the 'mixed' pathway open to you for longer; and early skin-to-skin and some breastfeeds at this stage will also help to lay down those foundations for you.

A change of direction after the birth

It is well-established that in the UK, at least 80% of women approach motherhood with the intention of breastfeeding their babies, and that this number drops by half in the first six weeks.[3] Of those who stopped breastfeeding by six weeks, nine out of 10 reported that they had planned to breastfeed for longer. Somewhere in these bleak statistics, we have those families where the original plan was exclusive breastfeeding, and formula has been introduced for one of the many reasons we have already discussed. And even though some breastfeeding is still happening, these mothers still have very mixed feelings about their situation.

'The "mum guilt" was awful. I felt like a failure and the

*extra worry about baby not latching properly afterwards,
and not being able to support my baby the way I should.'*
Stephanie

*'I was devastated at first but didn't have a choice.
Combination feeding is great for us. Not spoken about in
pregnancy at all.'* Alex

*'I knew it was the right decision, because my babies needed
it – the medical professionals and my own instincts were
saying so. But I also felt like I'd failed – I'm not used to
not being able to do things I set out to do.'* Hilary

*'It felt good, as soon as we did it baby was more settled
as wasn't hungry all the time so that made us all more
settled. A little guilty the first time until we saw the
effects.'* Louise

Grief and loss

If you are feeling guilt, anger, shock, disappointment, blaming
yourself, or telling yourself you have failed, you are not alone,
and you are not wrong to have these feelings. Breastfeeding has
been put on a pedestal for you, and then the barriers making it
hard to achieve have been stacked up. All of these feelings are
a normal part of grieving the loss of your expectation of what
motherhood would be like for you.

Breastfeeding is completely tied up with an ideal of
motherhood, portrayed in the media as both idyllic and
simultaneously unachievable; talked about with both envy
and contempt as the work of earth mothers, those to whom
mothering comes naturally, who probably had a home
waterbirth under the stars, who probably crochet their own

Why Mixed Feeding Matters

bread. Where are all these amazing women? I'm not sure they exist. In fact, breastfeeding is in the first instance a bodily function that nourishes babies, and knowing this but not being able to do it, is hard.

Throughout pregnancy, you are going through a transition to parenthood, and you have probably thought about what sort of mother you will be. To arrive in parent-land and find that it is not at all what you thought it would be like, takes some readjustment. Bereavement expert Kenneth Doka[4] calls this 'disenfranchised grief' – a grief or loss that is not publicly acknowledged, one that is often dismissed as 'at least you've got a healthy baby', or 'happy mum, happy baby', or 'fed is best'. It can be hard to be around people who seem to be finding breastfeeding easy, and it perhaps explains why you tend not to hear stories of straightforward breastfeeding. People know that if they were one of the lucky ones, they should not make a big deal about it. But perhaps if people did talk about straightforward breastfeeding a bit more, then this might come to feel more normal, more likely, more achievable.

'You did not fail. No woman 'fails' to breastfeed.
They are failed by a system that fails to support them,
both during breastfeeding and when they cannot.' Amy
Brown, *Why Breastfeeding Grief and Trauma Matter*[5]

Trauma when breastfeeding does not go as planned

'I was desperately sad feeling that I had failed her and couldn't do what should be natural to me. Talking about feeding or seeing other mums feeding without issues was a big trigger for me. I was also petrified that baby would get used to the bottle and reject the breast. This was by far

the hardest part of motherhood. People told me it really didn't matter but [...] I couldn't just take it.' Anna

Nowadays it is recognised that birth trauma is defined by the woman experiencing it, and on this basis, difficulties in breastfeeding can also be described as traumatic. Traumatic experiences include feeling that you or someone you love is in serious physical or psychological danger, and the anxiety of not feeling that you can feed your baby, or that you might damage them by giving them formula milk, certainly fits within this definition. Not feeling like you are being listened to or believed can also contribute to trauma, and if I had a pound for every mother who contacted me saying 'I've been told the latch is fine, but it's extremely painful and my nipples are getting damaged', then I would be able to pay for better breastfeeding support to help more families reach their goals. Yes, new mothers feel a lot of anxiety, and we have said above that a certain amount of doubt is a good thing – but that doesn't mean they don't deserve to be listened to with compassion and without judgement.

'I felt devastated.' Priya

Symptoms of trauma include intrusive or overwhelming thoughts or flashbacks, avoiding events that remind you of the trauma, negative thoughts and feelings including guilt and shame, and feelings of heightened arousal, such as irritability and difficulty in concentration. The duration and severity of these symptoms is key to diagnosis; many new mothers feel mild versions of these things, but if they are affecting your day-to-day life, then it is time to seek some help.

'I was sad reading things like "exclusive breastfeeding" stats because I knew we didn't count in them.' Hilary

Postnatal depression (PND)

There is a growing body of research telling us that when breastfeeding does not go to plan, this is associated with an increased risk of postnatal depression (See Borra et al, 2015,[6] among others, although interestingly this study found that mothers who had *not* planned to breastfeed, but did, were at the highest risk of PND). So far I have not found research that looks at what happens where *some* breastfeeding continues; that is, the mother goes on to use both breastmilk and formula. I would hypothesise that if this was a positive intention then continuing to breastfeed probably has some protective effect against PND, but where formula is introduced earlier than was planned, it may still contribute to PND. When I have found/done this research, I'll update the book.

Where mothers stop breastfeeding before they had planned to, this is often because they are experiencing pain or other difficulties.[7] Unfortunately, when mothers do experience pain and other difficulties with breastfeeding, they are quite likely to be advised to stop, with formula seen as the easy solution – which it is, if you define the problem as the baby not getting enough milk. But if a mother is experiencing pain or other difficulties with breastfeeding, then *she* might define the problem as the pain or the other difficulties, in which case that's what she needs support with. And if stopping before she is ready may contribute to postnatal depression, then advice to stop might not be the most helpful thing.

What to do with all these feelings

In the next chapter, I'll outline all the different people who might be able to support you with feeding your baby. For the specific things we have looked at in this chapter, including trauma and depression, there are some self-help strategies, as well as appropriate professional support, for you to try. Start, though, with acknowledging that this is how you feel, that your feelings are valid, and that you deserve help.

Self-help

If you already know that you are at risk of postnatal depression, then you can plan your support in advance, and this may take one thing off your list of worries. Here are some ideas to consider:

Friends and family can provide practical and emotional help, or you may need someone to manage their presence in your life, if you find them overwhelming. If you have a partner or someone else giving you close support, talk to them about what you need from them.

Mum and baby groups run by NCT, local children's centres, and other charities might help you to find your team. If turning up at one of these groups on your own feels like too big a step, you could ask someone to go with you, or you could contact the organiser and ask them to greet you at the door.

Online groups for new parents can be another way to find support, and sometimes these can connect you with local people whom you might eventually meet in real life.

Getting enough sleep is hard enough when you have a new baby, and can also be a factor in postnatal depression. If people are offering to help, as visitors to new families often do, think about whether this is something they could help with: can they take your baby while you sleep (or shower, or go for a run, etc)? Or if co-sleeping is an option that allows you to get more rest, can they be awake and watchful, if that gives you more confidence in this solution?

Talking about your feelings, whether about the birth, feeding, or becoming a parent, can be helpful. It may be that you have people in your life who will listen; I will also list the websites for some organisations below, which offer helplines staffed by trained volunteers.

Get some practical help, whether that's from your partner, your family, or those many other visitors, all of whom should be asking what they can do for you, otherwise why are you letting them in? If funds allow, then a cleaner or a postnatal doula might be what you need.

Get some exercise, because studies do show that this alleviates the symptoms of depression. This could be as low key as getting out for a walk with your baby in a sling. Or it might involve organising a helper to hold your baby while you get your dose of cold water swimming (or is that just me? In which case substitute yoga, gym class, a 5k run, etc). There are even mum and baby yoga classes that you can go to together.

Get professional help if your symptoms are serious or if you are in any way worried. In some areas you can self-refer to talking therapies; alternatively ask your health visitor or your GP to refer you. Again, if this feels like a big step, rope someone in to give you support.

Useful organisations

MIND www.mind.org.uk/information-support/types-of-
      mental-health-problems/postnatal-depression-and-
      perinatal-mental-health/self-care/
Tommy's www.tommys.org/pregnancy-information/im-
      pregnant/mental-health-wellbeing/postnatal-depression-pnd
PANDAS pandasfoundation.org.uk/
NCT www.nct.org.uk/

and Mia Scotland's excellent book, *Why Perinatal Depression Matters*, also published by Pinter & Martin.

10

Getting support with mixed feeding

As a breastfeeding counsellor, most of the parents I support are mixed feeding, and they don't call me because they are happy and finding things straightforward – they call me because they want something to change, whether that's the situation, or the way they feel about it. Over and over again while writing this book, I have found myself saying 'seek skilled breastfeeding support', and I am saying that one more time: find someone with breastfeeding knowledge, non-judgemental listening skills, and their own supportive network to back them up with situations that fall outside their experience.

A breastfeeding problem usually has a breastfeeding solution. Your job is to find the person who can help you to reach that solution, whether it's a solution that leads you towards more breastfeeding, or less. As a general rule, if you are asking for breastfeeding support and someone is telling you one of the following, then you have not yet asked the right person:

- the latch is fine (yet you are crying or in pain or there is visible damage)
- your only option is to express or to introduce some or more formula milk
- that once you have introduced formula there is no point in continuing to breastfeed
- that you must continue breastfeeding, whether or not you want to

'I felt pressured to stick to breast only to start, but I wanted my partner to share feeding responsibility.' Chloe

Sadness about breastfeeding stays with you. I still have moments of it, 16 years later. Sometimes when I meet a new person and they ask me what I do for a living, they tell me their own breastfeeding story, even if it's decades old. People remember how they felt, and if they had support, they remember feeling supported.

So who can help you?

Before the birth

You may have the opportunity to attend antenatal classes, whether that's a full course covering labour, birth and postnatal matters, or a standalone breastfeeding session. These are sometimes provided free by the NHS – ask your midwife if these are available in your area. There are also private providers, of which NCT is the best known and has the most extensive practitioner training. I say this with confidence as one of the practitioner trainers.

There are plenty of books and websites, though it can be tricky to untangle opinion from accurate fact online. Two of my colleagues and I have created a podcast called The Breastfeeding Show, available on Spotify and iTunes.

Straight after birth

If you have your baby in hospital, you are about to find out that every member of staff you meet has a small amount of breastfeeding training. This is the UNICEF Baby Friendly 18-hour training, which you can compare with training for breastfeeding counsellors and lactation consultants on the LCGB website here: lcgb.org/wp-content/uploads/2015/01/Whos-Who-in-Breastfeeding-in-the-UK-2014.pdf

What they often don't have is time to sit with every new mum and baby for as long as they need to really figure things out, and so occasionally they will resort to quick fixes such as pushing the baby's head on to the breast, or suggesting you express or give formula. If these are not things you are comfortable with, then you can ask for the *infant feeding team*, who are midwives with more specialist breastfeeding training. If you decide to use some formula or expressed milk, ask for help with paced bottle-feeding, or how to use a feeding cup (both explained in Chapter 5), and remember that some skilled breastfeeding support might also be needed, to help get the breastfeeding started, and keep the option of mixed feeding available to you.

Sometimes people feel pressured by midwives to start breastfeeding: midwives are aware of the factors that help to establish breastfeeding, and so will try to encourage you to feed early and have lots of skin-to-skin. Midwives also know how much difference it can make if early feeds go well, and it must be incredibly frustrating to work within a system that rarely allows them the time and mental space to really help new mothers with this.

You can also call in to one of the three *national breastfeeding helplines* (numbers at the end of this chapter) from the hospital; or if you have met a breastfeeding counsellor before the birth (e.g. at an antenatal class) you may be able to contact her directly.

If you have your baby at home, your midwife is likely to have more time to help you, or you may also have a doula present. *Doulas* are women with non-medical training who help at births and postnatally; they are often excellent sources of breastfeeding support, and sometimes are also qualified breastfeeding supporters.

In the days and weeks following the birth

You will usually be signed off from your midwife around 10–14 days after your baby's birth, after which your care comes under the community *health visiting team*. Like midwives, most health visitors will have a small amount of breastfeeding training, and occasionally you will meet one who has opted to specialise further. Most health visitors are not qualified to identify tongue ties or manage complex breastfeeding issues, but should know enough to signpost you to more specialist support.

GPs may have little or no specific training on breastfeeding,[1,2] and are likely only to see breastfeeding when it is problematic, meaning their knowledge can be a little skewed away from what's normal. There are some great resources available to them on the GP Infant Feeding Network website.

'I introduced formula earlier than I planned to, because of poor weight gain and pressure from health professionals without investigation into why. I felt sad, frustrated, unsupported, bullied.' Frankie

'My baby wasn't gaining as expected, and although there was obviously something wrong with milk transfer (she fed for over an hour per breast at 10 weeks and sometimes would not be satisfied) it was never diagnosed. I couldn't get out of the house because she started screaming for milk within 10 minutes of getting her in the pram.' Ali

Specialist breastfeeding support

> *'I wish I had known what support was out there (didn't know anything about peer supporters, lactation consultants etc!)'* Lara

Let me tell you about all the support that is out there. And let me remind you that a good breastfeeding supporter is as ready to support you to stop breastfeeding, to introduce a bottle, to express, to start solid foods, or to moan about how little sleep you are getting, as much as she is there to help you resolve any specific breastfeeding issues you may have.

Breastfeeding support groups

If you are lucky and still have an open Children's Centre near you, this is a good place to start. They may well have a baby clinic (where you would go to weigh your baby and talk to a health visitor), and sometimes offer breastfeeding support alongside this. The qualifications of the people offering that support can vary quite a lot, but it is at least a place where you might meet other new parents in a similar situation to you, to compare notes and get some company through the long afternoons of early motherhood.

There are four national breastfeeding charities, and a number of smaller local charities. Most of these offer breastfeeding support groups. The availability of these groups varies across the country, and is usually offered by breastfeeding counsellors (who may volunteer or have a grant-funded role) and volunteer breastfeeding peer supporters. They are usually free, and sometimes ask for donations or make a small charge for refreshments.

Breastfeeding peer supporters are usually mothers who have breastfed, and who have had around 20 hours of accredited training from one of the main breastfeeding charities. They should receive ongoing updates, and be insured by the accrediting body. Their training includes an understanding of normal breastfeeding, and listening skills. They should refer complex issues, including mixed feeding questions, on to a breastfeeding counsellor or other appropriate health professional.

Breastfeeding counsellors are mothers who have breastfed for at least six months, and will have had at least two years of part-time training in a range of breastfeeding subjects, as well as in non-judgemental counselling skills. This will – crucially – have allowed them the opportunity to debrief their own experience, so that they can offer you unbiased, parent-centred support. Breastfeeding counsellors work in voluntary and paid roles, and may spend a long time working alongside families, supporting them to navigate their infant feeding journeys. Different charities train their breastfeeding counsellors at different levels; NCT training is university accredited, the Breastfeeding Network designate their breastfeeding counsellors as 'Supporters' and the training is equivalent to an A-level, and training with the Association of Breastfeeding Mothers and La Leche League is largely online and self-directed. La Leche League designate their breastfeeding counsellors as 'Leaders'.

Lactation consultants come from either a health professional or a breastfeeding counsellor background, and so their personal experience of breastfeeding, and level of counselling skills, will vary accordingly. They need 1,000 hours of clinical experience, and then at least 90 hours of breastfeeding education covering complex and high-risk situations to qualify. Some are qualified to diagnose and treat tongue ties. They may work in paid roles in the NHS, and/or in private practice.

Twins and multiples: in Chapter 7, Janet Rimmer lists a number of sources of support for feeding twins and multiples.

Whoever you reach out to for support, it is always okay to trust your instincts, and ask for a second opinion if you need it. No breastfeeding supporter should be opposed to a team approach, perhaps with clinical support from one person, and listening and encouragement from another. All infant feeding supporters should be evidence-based, kind, and non-judgemental; and should know when to refer you to someone who can support you better than they can.

Useful organisations

NCT nct.org.uk

NCT Infant Feeding Line 0300 3300 700 option 1 8am-midnight every day

Association of Breastfeeding Mothers (ABM) abm.me.uk

Breastfeeding Network (BfN) breastfeedingnetwork.org.uk

National Breastfeeding Helpline 0300 100 0212 9.30am – 9.30pm

La Leche League GB laleche.org.uk 0345 120 2918 8am to 11pm

Lactation Consultants of Great Britain lcgb.org

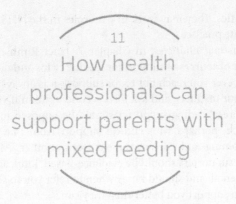

11

How health professionals can support parents with mixed feeding

I'm going to make the assumption that you, dear health professional, have read the rest of the book, despite being as thinly stretched for time and resources as I know you are. Maybe you already knew all that I have covered, which is brilliant; maybe some of it was new. If you feel like there are still some gaps in your knowledge, there are some great resources for you, which I'll list at the end of this chapter.

What do parents who are mixed feeding need from health professionals?

Parents very often want simple answers, and we know that this can be a rather tall order, because feeding situations can be so complex. This may result in families being given conflicting advice by the different health professionals they speak to, who may have responded to different questions at different times, without knowing what other people have said. This is so confusing and undermining to new parents' confidence.

'I felt really let down by some medical workers and they contradicted one another. I should have trusted myself more.' Becky

Why are they mixed feeding?

Parents use a mixture of breastmilk and formula for a huge number of individual reasons. In some cases this might feel like a positive decision that they have made and they are happy with, which does not mean they don't need support: continuing to breastfeed when formula is being used can be a challenge, and they will need an understanding of how to maintain the supply of breastmilk.

Formula might be used alongside breastmilk to address broader issues around needing support from partners and extended family, returning to work or education, tiredness, or embarrassment about breastfeeding in front of other people. Helping them work through these issues may be useful alongside offering or signposting to feeding support.

In my own review of the literature around mixed feeding, it was clear that parents were aware of positive health outcomes of breastfeeding, but were unconvinced that this was a long-term option. This was often because they understood breastfeeding to be difficult, restrictive, and had heard so many stories from women whose milk just dried up after two weeks; or because they believed the benefits to be time-limited – just a few weeks would be enough to give the baby the goodness of breastmilk – and breastmilk to be unreliable in terms of both supply and composition, subject to the mother's diet, stress levels and lifestyle. Formula, meanwhile, appears to be a stable, scientific product that promises to complement breastfeeding.

'I want her to have the formula too because it has vitamins, just in case.'[1]

The situation I have encountered the most often as a breastfeeding counsellor is where formula is being used alongside breastfeeding because of early breastfeeding issues. Parents are advised by health professionals to offer formula top-ups in the very early days, often with a recommendation to express breastmilk as well, and leave the postnatal ward with little idea of how to move forward from this convoluted position. There is no straightforward answer to preventing this from arising, or at least not one for which resources are readily available (skilled breastfeeding support on the postnatal ward, obviously), which means that health professionals in the community and voluntary breastfeeding supporters are left trying to pick up the threads and help parents to work out where to go from here.

Where to go from here

When you encounter a family using both breastmilk and formula, they are at a specific point on their journey, and it will be useful to establish their preferred direction of travel: do they want to move towards more breastfeeding or less breastfeeding, or do they need support to stay where they are? It is important to acknowledge to parents that it is possible to continue breastfeeding alongside using formula, and to support them with the information that will help them to do this.

Chapter 6 covers increasing and decreasing breastfeeding, and Chapter 2 covers what they will need to know to maintain the supply of breastmilk. However, each family really needs support tailored to their situation, their needs, and their hopes for the ongoing journey of feeding their baby.

When it comes to supporting parents with a combination of breastfeeding and bottle-feeding, there are often a lot of factors to take into account. It is worth having to hand the numbers for the main breastfeeding helplines so that you can offer these to families who need more time and attention to support them in their decision-making. There is no substitute for an in-depth knowledge of breastfeeding, counselling skills, and time to listen, and it's certainly better to acknowledge when you don't have all of these available to you, and signpost to someone who does.

> *'[I wish I had known] how emotionally challenging it is to receive such conflicting advice from medical professionals and that there is no one answer to a lot of things.'* Violet

Please do also look at Chapter 7, where Janet Rimmer has some suggestions for health professionals supporting parents of twins and multiples.

> *'My partner and family and friends were very supportive, healthcare professionals not so much. They didn't seem that well informed about [mixed feeding] as an option in my opinion. If you weren't exclusively breastfeeding it felt like you were a lost cause so might as well formula feed.'* Louise

Specialist support with infant feeding is available from
NCT nct.org.uk
NCT Infant Feeding Line 0300 3300 700 option 1 8am–midnight every day
Association of Breastfeeding Mothers (ABM) abm.me.uk
Breastfeeding Network (BfN) breastfeedingnetwork.org.uk
National Breastfeeding Helpline 0300 100 0212 9.30am – 9.30pm

La Leche League GB laleche.org.uk 0345 1202918 8am – 11pm

Lactation Consultants of Great Britain lcgb.org

Resources for health professionals

Banks, S. (2022) *Why Formula Feeding Matters* London: Pinter & Martin

Brown, A. (2019) *Informed Is Best* London: Pinter & Martin

Brown, A., (2018) 'What do women lose if they are prevented from meeting their breastfeeding goals?' *Clin Lactat* 9(4):200-7

Brown, A., & Jones, W. (eds) (2020) *A guide to supporting breastfeeding for the medical profession* London: Routledge

Breastfeeding and Medication – Dr Wendy Jones: breastfeeding-and-medication.co.uk/

The GP Infant Feeding Network: gpifn.org.uk/ *especially* the Guide to Essentials when supporting Breastfeeding Mothers, found here: gpifn.files.wordpress.com/2016/11/essential-guide-2017-web-version.pdf

First Steps Nutrition Trust: www.firststepsnutrition.org/infant-milks-health-workers

Kendall-Tackett, K. (2007) 'A new paradigm for depression in new mothers: the central role of inflammation and how breastfeeding and anti-inflammatory treatments protect maternal mental health.' *Int Breastfeed J* 2(1):6

National Library of Medicine's LactMed Database: www.ncbi.nlm.nih.gov/books/NBK501922/

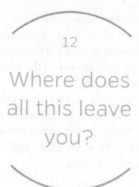

12

Where does all this leave you?

In writing this book, my aim was to demystify a lot of information about feeding babies, in order to make it easier for parents to make decisions. This was born out of my experience of working with parents and parents-to-be over the last 15 years, as well as the vast body of research that tells us how parents feel in those first weeks and months of the transition to parenthood, and how feeding decisions are so often a big part of those feelings: unprepared for the reality of life with a new baby, unsupported, judged, disappointed. I really hope that reading this has helped with even one of those things, and that you are able to access good quality support for the others.

I am concluding with some key messages from the book, a sort of easy-to-use guide for when you're feeling particularly frazzled.

You don't have to pick a side

Breastfeeding and formula feeding are not all-or-nothing behaviours. Any amount of breastmilk will benefit your baby, and any amount of breastfeeding or expressing keeps the door open just a chink for increasing that, if you want to.

Furthermore, you never have to explain or justify your decisions to anyone. You deserve the same amount of accurate, patient, non-judgemental support as the next mum, no matter how they are feeding their baby.

And finally, on this subject, very often your decisions don't need to be final. You can, for example, make a plan for the rest of this week, and then review it. If you reduce the amount of breastfeeding, then (with some effort and support), you can increase it again; and vice versa.

> '[It helped that] the consultant at the hospital was really kind and emphasised that the feeding plan was aiming to get back to breastfeeding if that's what I wanted. Ready-mixed formula helped practically as I only did it for two weeks then was told to focus on breastfeeding and building my supply.' Sarah

For mixed feeding to be an option, breastfeeding needs to work

This means it can be most helpful to focus on breastfeeding first, and introduce other means of feeding your baby once you feel comfortable that it is working. If you don't have the luxury of doing this, then be aware of the tools you have for protecting your breastmilk supply (namely expressing, skin-to-skin, and offering breastfeeds as often as possible even if they feel short and ineffective).

It doesn't matter which brand of formula you use; they are all the same

It does need to be first infant formula, and you do need to prepare it safely according to the instructions.

Expressing is a bit of a mixed blessing

Expressing in addition to breastfeeding can increase the overall supply of milk. Expressing instead of breastfeeding can decrease it. Expressing is a wonderful thing that you can do to help your baby get breastmilk, in all sorts of difficult circumstances, but it is also an additional chore to add to your busy day.

You can bottle-feed in a responsive way

Many people want to use both breast and bottle to provide a bonding experience for the parent who isn't breastfeeding, so do make sure that you make this an interactive experience, responding to your baby's feeding cues, keeping them close when you feed them, and maintaining eye contact.

Maintaining breastfeeding alongside using formula, or expressing, is a balancing act

Some families get into a nice rhythm; others can find that the balance tips more heavily than they would like, one way or another. Generally speaking, it is more problematic where it's tipping towards formula use before the family is ready for that. If you're doing all three methods of feeding, then you may feel that you have a lot on your plate; this is not usually a sustainable long-term arrangement.

There is support out there for you

Anyone who supports breastfeeding should be non-judgemental and evidence-based, and if that's not what you're finding, I hope you can find an alternative source of support. And I will reiterate what I have said above: you never need to explain or justify your feeding decisions. There is more detail about what to expect from different types of breastfeeding

145

supporter on p136.

> *'[I wish I had known] how much support was out there*
> *for breastfeeding.'* Samira

Many, many parents struggle with different aspects of feeding their babies; you are not alone. Expressing, and using formula, are respectively the third and fourth most common reasons for calling the NCT Feeding Line, making up nearly half of all calls. So please don't feel that you can't ask for help with anything that you are finding hard, whether it's a straightforward question about something technical, or you have a lot of feelings to unload.

If you are looking for support, remember to check that the person you are contacting has appropriate training for what you need. There is no substitute for skilled support from someone who has the time to really listen to you, and the knowledge base to help out with whatever you need.

Finally

Whether you have read (or flicked through) this book before the birth of your baby, or you are in the thick of trying to figure out what to do next, I hope it has clarified some things for you. There is rarely one approach that will work for everyone, but if you understand how things work and are aware of what factors you need to take into consideration, you are well on your way to adapting the information I've given you to your own personal circumstances. Remember that you and your baby are doing the very best you can with what you've got, and that help is out there to support you to change the things that aren't working for you.

Acknowledgements

My friend and colleague Janet Rimmer initially agreed to write this with me, and then decided only to do the chapter on twins and multiples, for which she is supremely qualified. I am grateful to Janet for other things too, including her endless kindness and empathy. For me, WWJD means 'What would Janet do?'

Louise Oliver and Gillian Denton both contributed their experience and knowledge to the chapter on the neonatal unit. Louise went on to review some chapters and make really intelligent suggestions.

My NCT tutors, colleagues, and supervision group, who continue to shape the Breastfeeding Counsellor and the person I am. And all the parents I have ever supported, before and after their babies arrived, who have taught me so much about the value of non-judgemental listening and support.

Members of the NCT Wokingham Facebook group who shared their experiences and feelings, and are quoted throughout the book. Names have been changed as requested.

I have always wanted to write a book, so I was delighted when Martin Wagner agreed that I could write this one. Martin has been supporting my work for years. I can't believe it took him so long.

Most importantly of all, Frances Attenborough and Megan Stephenson, my friends, fellow BFCs, and the other two members of The Breastfeeding Show podcast team. You supported this project from the start; then read, commented on, and corrected my first draft. You are the shared set of evidence and empathy. Most of these words are as much yours as mine. Thank you.

References

Introduction

1. McAndrew F et al 2012 'Infant Feeding Survey 2010' Leeds: Health and Social Care Information Centre
2. Brown, A 2019 *Why Breastfeeding Grief and Trauma Matter* London: Pinter & Martin
3. Paul, L.A. (2014) *Transformative Experience* Oxford: OUP.
4. Brown, A 2016 What Do Women Really Want? Lessons for Breastfeeding Promotion and Education. *Breastfeed Med.* 2016 Apr;11:102-10. doi: 10.1089/bfm.2015.0175.
5. Burton, A 2022 A qualitative exploration of mixed-feeding in first-time mothers *British Journal of Midwifery* Jan 2022, 20-29
6. Woollard, F. (2018)Should we talk about the 'benefits' of breastfeeding? The significance of the default in representations of infant feeding *Journal of Medical Ethics* 2018;44:756-760.

1. Why do parents use both breastmilk and formula?

1. Victora, C. G et al 2016 Breastfeeding in the 21st century: epidemiology, mechanisms, and lifelong effect. *Lancet* (London, England), 387(10017), 475–490. https://doi.org/10.1016/S0140-6736(15)01024-7
2. Renfrew, M.J. et al 2012 *Preventing disease and saving resources: the potential contribution of increasing breastfeeding rates in the UK.* Unicef UK
3. Bryder, L. Breastfeeding and health professionals in Britain, New Zealand and the United States, 1900--1970. *Med Hist.* 2005 Apr;49(2):179-96.
4. WHO Code of Marketing of Breastmilk Substitutes. Unicef
5. Save The Children 2018 *Don't Push It: Why the formula industry needs to clean up its act.*
6. Burton, A. et al 2022 A qualitative exploration of mixed feeding intentions in first-time mothers *British Journal of Midwifery* Jan 2022 30:1
7. Baby Sleep Information Source (undated) *Normal Sleep Development* basisonline.org.uk
8. Galland, B.C. 2012. Normal sleep patterns in infants and children: a systematic review of observational studies. *Sleep medicine reviews*, 16(3), 213–222. https://doi.org/10.1016/j.smrv.2011.06.001
9. Rudzik, A.E.F., Ball, H.L. 2016 Exploring Maternal Perceptions of Infant

Sleep and Feeding Method Among Mothers in the United Kingdom: A Qualitative Focus Group Study. *Matern Child Health J.* Jan;20(1):33-40. doi: 10.1007/s10995-015-1798-7. PMID: 26156828.

10. Bartick, M. et al 2018 Babies in boxes and the missing links on safe sleep: Human evolution and cultural revolution *Matern Child Nutr.* 2018;14:e12544.

11. Fu, X., Lovell, A.L., Braakhuis, A.J., Mithen, R.F., Wall, C.R. 2021 Type of Milk Feeding and Introduction to Complementary Foods in Relation to Infant Sleep: A Systematic Review. *Nutrients.* 2021 Nov 16;13(11):4105

12. Montgomery-Downs, H.E., Clawges, H.M., Santy, E.E. 2010 Infant feeding methods and maternal sleep and daytime functioning. *Pediatrics.* 2010 Dec;126(6):e1562-8. doi: 10.1542/peds.2010-1269.

13. Doan, T., Gay, C.L., Kennedy, H.P., Newman, J., Lee, K.A. 2014 Nighttime breastfeeding behavior is associated with more nocturnal sleep among first-time mothers at one month postpartum. *J Clin Sleep Med.* 2014 Mar 15;10(3):313-9. doi: 10.5664/jcsm.3538. PMID: 24634630; PMCID: PMC3927438.

14. Hookway, L. 2020 *Let's Talk About Your New Family's Sleep* London: Pinter & Martin

15. Sacks, A. 2018 A new way to think about the transition to motherhood. YouTube https://www.youtube.com/watch?v=jOsX_HnJtHU

16. Godinez, L. (undated) *Fathers, Breastfeeding and Bonding* Breastfeeding Centre of Pittsburgh http://breastfeedingcenterofpittsburgh.com/bf101/fathers-breastfeeding-and-bonding/

17. Machin, A. 2018 *The Life of Dad* London: Simon & Schuster

18. Arbour, M.W. and Kessler, J.L. 2013 Mammary Hypoplasia: Not Every Breast Can Produce Sufficient Milk. *Journal of Midwifery & Women's Health*, 58: 457-461.

2: What do parents need to know about breastfeeding?

1. Parry, J.E., Ip DKM, Chau, P.Y.K., Wu, K.M., Tarrant, M. 2013 Predictors and Consequences of In-Hospital Formula Supplementation for Healthy Breastfeeding Newborns. *Journal of Human Lactation.* 2013;29(4):527-536

2. Caroline J. Chantry, Kathryn G. Dewey, Janet M. Peerson, Erin A. Wagner, Laurie A. Nommsen-Rivers 2014, In-Hospital Formula Use Increases Early Breastfeeding Cessation Among First-Time Mothers Intending to Exclusively Breastfeed, *The Journal of Pediatrics*, Volume

164, Issue 6, 2014, Pages 1339-1345.e5

3. Uvnäs Moburg, K. 2011 *The Oxytocin Factor* London: Pinter & Martin

4. Weissbluth, L., Weissbluth, M. 1992 Infant colic: the effect of serotonin and melatonin circadian rhythms on the intestinal smooth muscle. *Med Hypotheses.* 1992 Oct;39(2):164-7

5. NHS 2020 *Your baby's height and weight.* https://www.nhs.uk/conditions/baby/babys-development/height-weight-and-reviews/baby-height-and-weight/

3: What do parents need to know about using formula milk?

1. Brown, A., Lee, M. 2011 An exploration of the attitudes and experiences of mothers in the United Kingdom who chose to breastfeed exclusively for 6 months postpartum. *Breastfeed.Med* 2011;6:197-204.

2. Lee, E. 2007 Health, morality, and infant feeding: British mothers' experiences of formula milk use in the early weeks. *Sociology of Health and Illness* 2007;29(7):1075-90.

3. Lakshman, R., Ogilvie, D., Ong, K. 2009 Mothers' experiences of bottlefeeding: a systematic review of qualitative and quantitative studies. *Arch Dis Child* 2009;94(8):596-601

4. Brown, A., Jones, S.W., Evans, E. 2020 Marketing of infant milk in the UK: what do parents see and believe? *A report for First Steps Nutrition Trust.* London: First Steps Nutrition Trust

5. Channel 4 2019 *Dispatches: The Great Formula Milk Scandal* https://www.unicef.org.uk/babyfriendly/dispatches-great-formula-milk-scandal/

6. First Steps Nutrition (2022) *Costs of infant formula, follow-on formula and milks marketed as foods for special medical purposes available over the counter in the UK*

7. https://infantmilkinfo.org/wp-content/uploads/2022/04/Costs-of-IF-FOF-and-milks-marketed-as-FSMP-available-over-the-counter-in-the-UK_April2022.pdf

8. First Steps Nutrition Trust *Ingredients in infant milks - Protein content of infant milks report* https://static1.squarespace.com/static/59f75004f09ca48694070f3b/t/5e844ec4a5dfdd3303ea44dc/1585729220743/Protein_content_of_infant_milks.pdf

9. NHS (2019) *Types of Formula* https://www.nhs.uk/conditions/baby/breastfeeding-and-bottle-feeding/bottle-feeding/types-of-formula/

10. Organic milk: https://infantmilkinfo.org/wp-content/uploads/2021/09/Organic-formula_milk_FAQfinalfinal.pdf

4: What do parents need to know about expressing breastmilk?

1. Maternity Action 2002 *Continuing to breastfeed when you return to work* https://maternityaction.org.uk/advice/continuing-to-breastfeed-when-you-return-to-work/

2. NHS 2019 *Expressing and Storing Breastmilk* https://www.nhs.uk/conditions/baby/breastfeeding-and-bottle-feeding/breastfeeding/expressing-breast-milk/

5: What do parents need to know about using bottles and other feeding devices?

1. Maxwell, C., Fleming, K.M., Fleming, V., Porcellato, L. 2020 UK mothers' experiences of bottle refusal by their breastfed baby. *Matern Child Nutr.* 16:e13047. https://doi.org/10.1111/mcn.13047

2. McLeod, S 2021 *Object Permanence* Simply Psychology website https://www.simplypsychology.org/Object-Permanence.html

6: Managing breastfeeding alongside using formula

1. Crenshaw, J.T. 2019 Healthy Birth Practice #6: Keep Mother and Newborn Together-It's Best for Mother, Newborn, and Breastfeeding. *J Perinat Educ.* 2019 Apr 1;28(2):108-115

2. Bonyata, K. 2018 My expressed breastmilk doesn't smell fresh. What can I do? *Kellymom* https://kellymom.com/bf/pumpingmoms/milkstorage/lipase-expressedmilk/

3. NHS 2019 *Formula Milk: Common Questions* https://www.nhs.uk/conditions/baby/breastfeeding-and-bottle-feeding/bottle-feeding/formula-milk-questions/

4. Jones, W. 2017 *Why Mothers Medication Matters* London: Pinter & Martin

5. Jones, W. 2019 *Domperidone and Breastfeeding* Breastfeeding Network website *https://www.breastfeedingnetwork.org.uk/domperidone/*

7: Mixed feeding twins and multiples

1. Multiple Births Foundation (2011) Guidance for health professionals on feeding twins, triplets and higher order multiples https://www.multiplebirths.org.uk/assets/downloads/guidance-for-health-professionals-on-feeding-twins-triplets-and-hIgher-order-multiples.pdf

2. La Leche League GB My baby needs more milk https://www.laleche.org.uk/my-baby-needs-more-milk/

3. Unicef (2021) Building a happy baby: A guide for parents https://www.unicef.org.uk/babyfriendly/baby-friendly-resources/relationship-building-resources/building-a-happy-baby/

4. NHS (2021) Guide to bottle-feeding https://www.unicef.org.uk/babyfriendly/wp-content/uploads/sites/2/2008/02/start4life_guide_to_bottle_-feeding.pdf

5. HFEA (2022) Multiple births in fertility treatment 2019

6. https://www.hfea.gov.uk/about-us/publications/research-and-data/multiple-births-in-fertility-treatment-2019/#main-points

7. HFEA (2020) Family formations in fertility treatment 2018 https://www.hfea.gov.uk/about-us/publications/research-and-data/family-formations-in-fertility-treatment-2018/#mainpoints

8. NHS (2019) Pregnant with twins https://www.nhs.uk/pregnancy/finding-out/pregnant-with-twins/

9. NICE (2019) Twin and triplet guidance pregnancy https://www.nice.org.uk/guidance/ng137

10. Bradshaw et al, 2022 Risk factors associated with postpartum depressive symptoms: A multinational study *Journal of Affective Disorders* Vol 301 pp. 345-351

11. Moreton, C. (2020) The power of three https://www.bbc.co.uk/sounds/play/m000q26r

8: Mixed feeding and the neonatal unit

1. Bashir, T., Reddy, K.V., Kiran, S., Murki, S., Kulkarni, D., & Dinesh, P. 2019. Effect of colostrum given within the 12 hours after birth on feeding outcome, morbidity and mortality in very low birth weight infants: a prospective cohort study. *Sudanese Journal of Paediatrics,* 19(1), 19–24. https://doi.org/10.24911/SJP.106-1540825552

2. Gidrewicz, D.A., Fenton, T.R. (2014) A systematic review and meta-analysis of the nutrient content of preterm and term breast milk. *BMC Pediatr* 14, 216

3. Nolan, L.S.; Parks, O.B.; Good, M. A 2020 Review of the Immunomodulating Components of Maternal Breast Milk and Protection Against Necrotizing Enterocolitis. *Nutrients, 12,* 14. https://doi.org/10.3390/nu12010014

4. Morton, J., Hall, J., Wong, R. et al. 2009 Combining hand techniques with electric pumping increases milk production in mothers of preterm infants. *J Perinatol* 29, 757–764

5. Segal, F. 2019 *Mothership* London: Random House

9: Mixed feelings about mixed feeding

1. NCT (2018) Infant Feeding Message Framework
2. Stadlen, N. (2004) *What Mothers Do* London: Piatkus
3. McAndrew, F. et al 2012 'Infant Feeding Survey 2010' Leeds: Health and Social Care Information Centre
4. Doka, K.J. (2008). Disenfranchised grief in historical and cultural perspective. In M.S. Stroebe, R.O. Hansson, H. Schut, & W. Stroebe (Eds.), *Handbook of bereavement research and practice: Advances in theory and intervention* (pp.223–240). American Psychological Association
5. Brown, A. (2019) *Why breastfeeding grief and trauma matter* London: Pinter & Martin
6. Borra, C., Iacovou, M., & Sevilla, A. (2015). New evidence on breastfeeding and postpartum depression: the importance of understanding women's intentions. *Maternal and Child Health Journal*, 19(4), 897-907.
7. McAndrew, F. et al 2012 'Infant Feeding Survey 2010' Leeds: Health and Social Care Information Centre

10: Getting support with mixed feeding

1. Santhanam, L. (2019) GP Education GP Infant Feeding Network (UK) website
2. https://gpifn.org.uk/gp-education/
3. Santhanam, L. (2016) What do GPs know about breastfeeding? A Q&A with the GP Infant Feeding Network (part 1) *Parenting Science Gang blog* http://parentingsciencegang.org.uk/web-chats/what-do-gps-know-about-breastfeeding-a-qa-with-the-gp-infant-feeding-network-part-1/

11: How Health Professionals can support with mixed feeding

1. Bunik, M., Clark, L., Zimmer, L.M., Jimenez, L.M., O'Connor, M.E., Crane, L.A., & Kempe, A. (2006). Early infant feeding decisions in low-income Latinas. *Breastfeeding Medicine*, 1(4), 225-235. https://doi.org/10.1089/bfm.2006.1.225

Available from Pinter & Martin
in the Why it Matters series

Series editor: Susan Last

pinterandmartin.com